Biostatistics in Public Health Using STATA

Erick L. Suárez
Cynthia M. Pérez
Graciela M. Nogueras
Camille Moreno-Gorrín

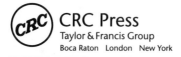

CRC Press
Taylor & Francis Group
Boca Raton   London   New York

CRC Press is an imprint of the
Taylor & Francis Group, an **informa** business

CRC Press
Taylor & Francis Group
6000 Broken Sound Parkway NW, Suite 300
Boca Raton, FL 33487-2742

© 2016 by Taylor & Francis Group, LLC
CRC Press is an imprint of Taylor & Francis Group, an Informa business

No claim to original U.S. Government works

Printed on acid-free paper
Version Date: 20160201

International Standard Book Number-13: 978-1-4987-2199-8 (Hardback)

Visit the Taylor & Francis Web site at
http://www.taylorandfrancis.com

and the CRC Press Web site at
http://www.crcpress.com

To our loved ones

To those who have enlightened our path throughout their knowledge.

Contents

Preface

This book is intended to serve as a guide to applied statistical analysis in public health using the Stata program. Our motivation for writing this book lies in our years of experience teaching biostatistics and epidemiology, particularly in the academic programs of biostatistics and epidemiology. The academic material is usually covered in biostatistics courses at the master's and doctoral levels at schools of public health. The main focus of this book is the application of statistics in public health. Because of its user-friendliness, we used the Stata software package in the creation of the database and the statistical analysis that will be seen herein. This 12-chapter book can serve equally well as a textbook or as a source for consultation. Readers will be exposed to the following topics: *Basic Commands, Data Description, Graph Construction, Significance Tests, Linear Regression Models, Analysis of Variance, Categorical Data Analysis, Logistic Regression Model, Poisson Regression Model, Survival Analysis, Analysis of Correlated Data,* and *Advanced Programming in Stata.* Each chapter is based on one or more research problems linked to public health. We have started with the assumption that the readers of this book have taken at least a basic course in biostatistics and epidemiology. Further, for those readers who are new to Stata, the first three chapters should be read sequentially, as they form the basis of an introductory course to this software.

Erick L. Suárez
University of Puerto Rico

Cynthia M. Pérez
University of Puerto Rico

Graciela M. Nogueras
MD Anderson Cancer Center

Camille Moreno-Gorrín
University of Puerto Rico

Acknowledgments

We thank Dr. Kenneth Hess, professor of biostatistics at MD Anderson Cancer Center in Houston, Texas, for his kind comments and suggestions aimed at improving different aspects of this book. We also thank Bob Ritchie for his excellent work in editing this book. We want to acknowledge the support we received from the Department of Biostatistics and Epidemiology of the Graduate School of Public Health, University of Puerto Rico, in the writing of this book. We are very grateful to the many students—particularly Marc Machín and Kristy Zoé Vélez of the MPH program in Biostatistics—who collaborated by reading material for this book.

This book would not have been possible without the financial support that we received from the following grants: CA096297/CA096300 from the National Cancer Institute of the National Institutes of Health and 2U54MD00758 from the National Institute on Minority Health and Health Disparities of the National Institutes of Health.

Authors

Erick L. Suárez is a professor of biostatistics in the Department of Biostatistics and Epidemiology at the University of Puerto Rico Graduate School of Public Health. He has more than 25 years of experience teaching biostatistics at the graduate level and has co-authored more than 75 peer-reviewed publications in chronic and infectious diseases. Dr. Suárez has been a co-investigator of several NIH-funded grants related to cancer, HPV, HCV, and diabetes. He has extensive experience in statistical consulting with biomedical researchers, particularly in the analysis of microarrays data in breast cancer.

Cynthia M. Pérez is a professor of epidemiology in the Department of Biostatistics and Epidemiology at the University of Puerto Rico Graduate School of Public Health. She has taught epidemiology and biostatistics for over 20 years. She has also directed efforts in mentoring and training to public health and medical students at the University of Puerto Rico. She has been the principal investigator or co-investigator of research grants in diverse areas of public health including diabetes, metabolic syndrome, periodontal disease, viral hepatitis, and HPV infection. She is the author or co-author of more than 75 peer-reviewed publications.

Graciela M. Nogueras is a statistical analyst at the University of Texas MD Anderson Cancer Center in Houston, Texas. She is currently enrolled on the PhD program in biostatistics at the University of Texas—Graduate School of Public Health. She has co-authored more than 30 peer-reviewed publications. For the past nine years, she has been performing statistical analyses for clinical and basic science researchers. She has been assisting with the design of clinical trials and animal research studies, performing sample size calculations, and writing the clinical trial reports of clinical trial progress and interim analyses of efficacy and safety data to the University of Texas MD Anderson Data and Safety Monitoring Board.

Camille Moreno-Gorrín is a graduate of the Master of Science Program in Epidemiology at the University of Puerto Rico Graduate School of Public Health. During her graduate studies, she was a research assistant at the Comprehensive Cancer Center of the University of Puerto Rico where she co-authored several articles in biomedical journals. She also worked as a research coordinator for the HIV/AIDS Surveillance System of the Puerto Rico Department of Health, where she conducted research on intervention programs to link HIV patients to care.

Chapter 1

Basic Commands

Aim: Upon completing the chapter, the learner should be able to understand the general form of the basic commands of Stata for reading and saving databases.

1.1 Introduction

Stata is a computer program designed to perform various statistical procedures. Among the basic statistical procedures that can be performed are the following: calculation of summary measures, construction of graphs, and frequency distribution using contingency tables. Furthermore, using Stata, you can perform parameter estimation in generalized linear models and survival analysis models using uncorrelated and correlated data. The program also has the ability to perform arithmetic operations on matrices. Its ability to export and import databases in the Excel format gives Stata great versatility. This program is regularly used in biostatistics courses in public health schools in different countries. It is also often cited as one of the main programs used for statistical analysis in scientific publications related to public health research.

This chapter will provide an introduction to the Stata program, version 14.0. We assume that readers of this book have a basic knowledge of both biostatistics and epidemiology.

1.2 Entering Stata

After selecting the Stata icon on your computer, the program responds with five windows (Figure 1.1), which have the following utilities:

1. *Command*: In this window the user can write or enter "commands" or instructions to perform various operations with an active database. Not all commands can be executed in this area; there is also a taskbar with executable commands.
2. *Results*: This window shows the results obtained after the execution of the commands introduced or requested via the taskbar.
3. *Variables*: In this window the variables of an active database are displayed. If this window is blank, that is an indication that there is no active database.
4. *Review*: This window lists all the commands used during the current open session of the program and allows them to be repeated without rewriting them in the command area.
5. *Properties*: This window displays the properties of the user's variables and dataset.

1.3 Taskbar

The taskbar provides common access to all windows-based program commands, such as *File*, *Edit*, *Data*, *Graphics*, and *Statistics*; these options can be found at the upper part of the main window. The most frequently used icon is the *Data Editor* icon, with which

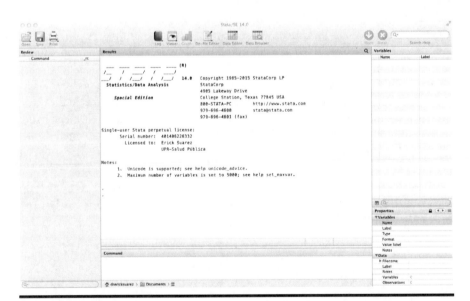

Figure 1.1 Main Stata 14 window.

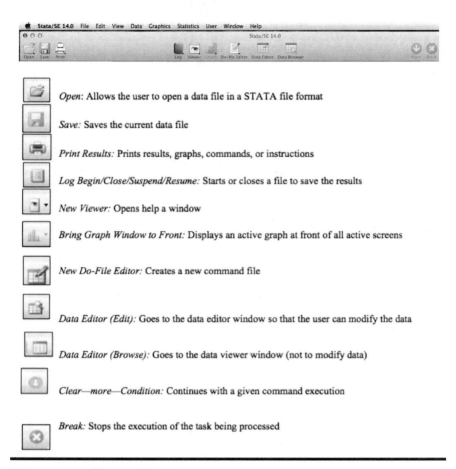

Figure 1.2   Taskbar and icons.

it is possible to enter values and identify the variables in a given project. The *Graphics* button provides access to the window used to generate different types of graphs. The *Statistics* option allows the user to perform statistical mathematical operations through the execution of the commands. Below the taskbar are icons that allow the user to open, save, and print, along with icons that facilitate the observation of graphics (Figure 1.2).

1.4 Help

One of the most useful attributes of Stata is its support system, which allows the user to find the commands and their ways of execution, according to that user's specific needs. The help menu can be accessed by clicking on the "New Viewer" icon on the toolbar or by typing either *help* or the letter *h* in the command area and following that with a keyword that represents the topic about which the user requires more information (see Figure 1.3).

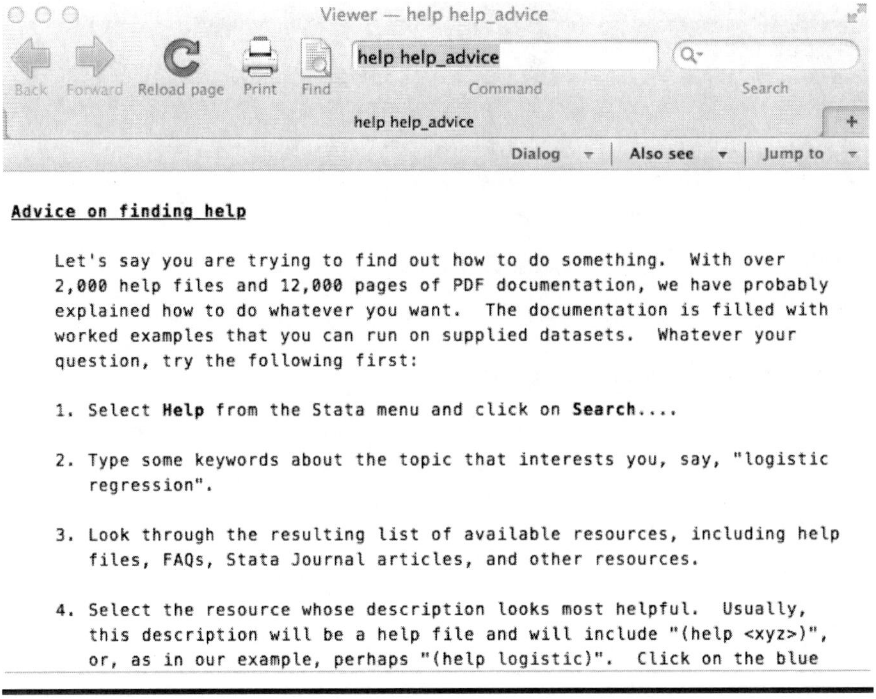

Figure 1.3   Help window.

For example, if we want to learn how to perform an analysis of variance (ANOVA), we can use one of the following commands:

```
help anova
```

or

```
h anova
```

Upon entering those commands, a specific window for ANOVA will appear (see Figure 1.4).

1.5 Stata Working Directories

When working with Stata, files and results can be saved to a specific directory, which is defined during the installation instructions. For example, to view the working directory for a project, enter the command *pwd* (*p*ath of the current *w*orking *d*irectory), and the following results will be displayed:

```
. pwd
  /Users/Documents/students
```

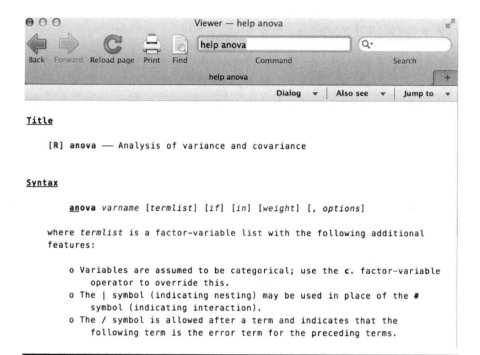

Figure 1.4   Help ANOVA.

It is important to keep the working files in a directory that is different from the default directory that Stata assigns, because during the regular program updates files located in the default directory may be removed.

To create a particular file, the *mkdir* and *cd* commands must be used to navigate to that directory again. The sequence of commands to create a directory is as follows:

cd C:\	Navigate to the main directory of your hard drive or to the location where you wish to create your home directory
mkdir new_folder	Create a new working directory
cd new_folder	Navigate to the new working directory

To use Stata in the new working directory, you need to restart the program and immediately move to the desired directory. For example, assuming that the name of the working directory is "students" and assuming, as well, that this directory is located in your computer's *Documents* folder, the following will take you to that folder:

```
cd "/Users/Documents/students"
```

1.6 Reading a Data File

After creating the working directory in which, outside the Stata program, we have previously copied a data file (i.e., the file named "Cancer.dta"), we proceed to open the file. This can be done in two different ways: using the command area or using the icon on the toolbar. For the former, we would write the following command sequence:

cd "C:\new_folder" dir use cancer	Command to navigate to the new working directory Command to browse the contents of the folder The **use** command indicates the name of the file that will be used

For the latter, on the other hand, it is necessary to click , the *Open* icon, and browse the folder that contains the working file. The ***describe*** command can be used to view the information contained in the data file, which might include the number of observations, variables, and file size, among others, as shown below (assuming that the active database being used contains the anthropometric measurements of 10 subjects):

```
describe
```

Output

```
. describe

Contains data
  obs:           10
  vars:           5
  size:         200
------------------------------------------------------------------------
              storage   display    value
variable name   type     format    label      variable label
------------------------------------------------------------------------
var1            float    %9.0g
var2            float    %9.0g
var3            float    %9.0g
var4            float    %9.0g
var5            float    %9.0g
------------------------------------------------------------------------
```

1.7 *insheet* Procedure

Another way to read a database in Stata is to import existing databases created in other formats. Delimited text files using the .txt (can be opened by most text editors), .raw (a raw image file), and .csv (an MS Excel file) extensions can be imported into Stata. The most commonly used is .csv, which, as indicated, is created using MS Excel. In Excel, you must save the data file using the .csv file extension instead of the .xls extension. When you have the data saved with .csv, you can then proceed to use the *insheet* command in Stata:

```
insheet using "c:/data.csv", replace
```

The *replace* option that has been placed after the comma (above) is used to clear the program if another database was being used. Stata does not open a database if there is another one that is already open. The *clear* command can also be used in Stata to remove a database, therefore clearing the way to use a new one.

1.8 Types of Files

Below is a list of the different types of archives that can be created in Stata; the left-hand column contains the file extensions that correspond to each archive.

.dta	data files
.do	command files
.ado	programs
.hlp	help files
.gph	graphs
.dct	dictionary files

1.9 Data Editor

In the Data Editor window, you can input data for the creation and identification of the study variables. One advantage of Stata's data editor is its ability to import databases built in Excel. This is done by the simple operation of selecting the entire database in Excel and copying and pasting it into the Stata data editor.

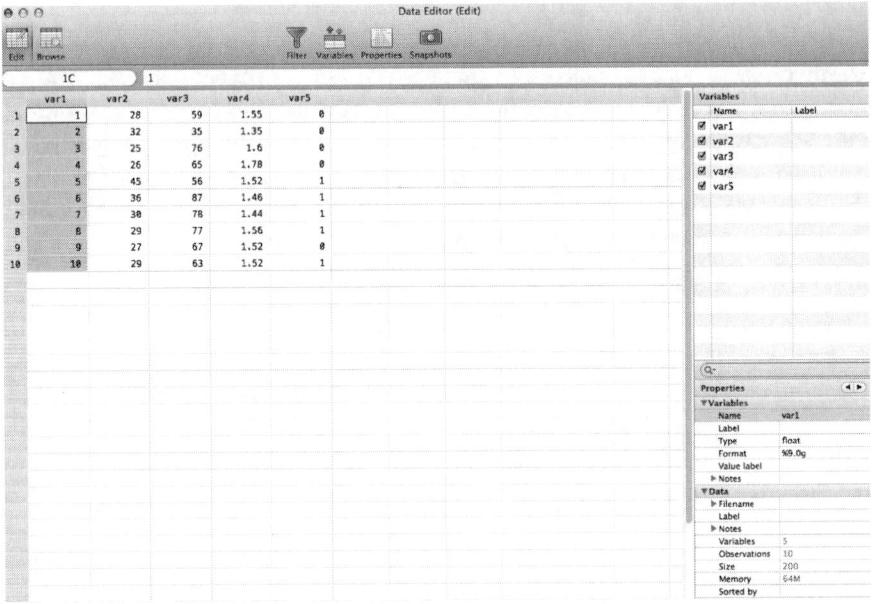

Figure 1.5   Data Editor window.

To access the Data Editor window (Figure 1.5), click the "Edit" icon, , on the taskbar located in the main window.

At the beginning of the data entry process, the program automatically assigns a name to the column that defines each variable (var1, var2, …, vark). This name can be changed in the Variables Manager window after clicking the *Data Editor* icon, using the box "Name" (Figure 1.6). To return to the main window of Stata, you close or minimize the Data Editor window.

Constructing a user-friendly database requires that each variable be named in such a way as to be easy to identify. This can be done using the "Label" box in the properties window. When building a database, it is possible for the values assigned to the variables to be represented by codes. The coding of the variables can be done using the "Value Label" option. With this option you can assign numerical values to alpha-numeric variables, thereby allowing better management of the database. This coding can be done in the Variables Manager window. The steps to do this are as follows:

1. Click "Manage" in the *Variables Manager* window, and a new window appears (Figure 1.7). Then click "Create Label" to assign each code a label.
2. After creating the value labels, return to the *Variables Manager* window, in which you will be able to assign labels to each variable in the "Label" box (if they were not assigned previously in the *Properties* window) (Figure 1.8).

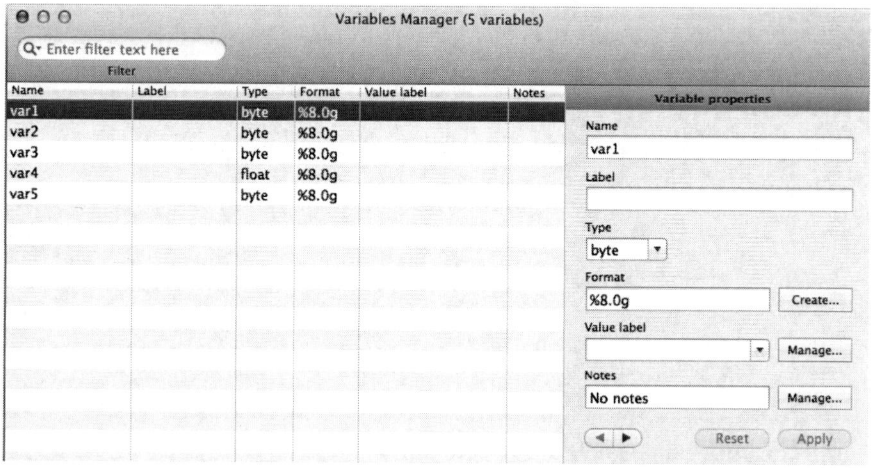

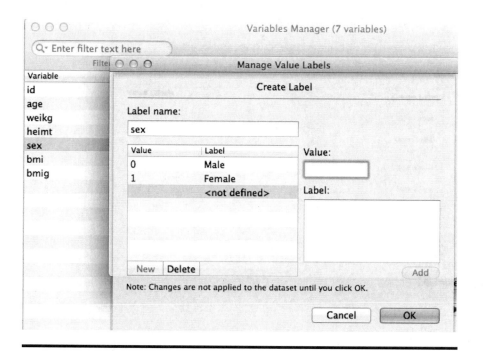

Figure 1.6   Variable name change.

Figure 1.7   Assigning value label.

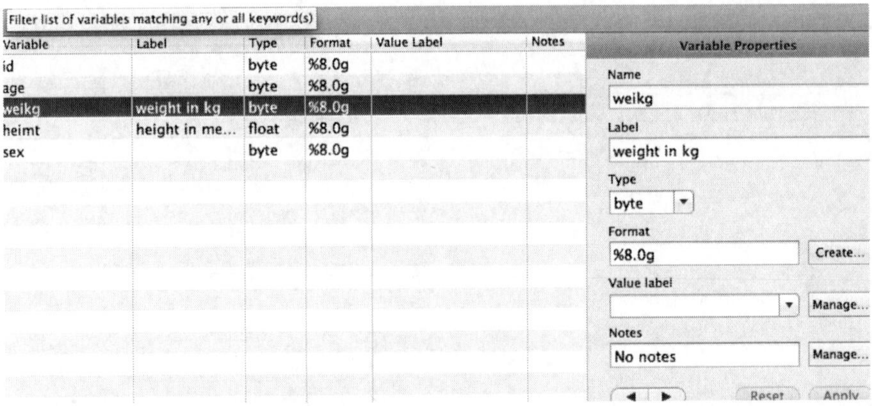

Variable	Label	Type	Format	Value Label	Notes
id		byte	%8.0g		
age		byte	%8.0g		
weikg	weight in kg	byte	%8.0g		
heimt	height in me...	float	%8.0g		
sex		byte	%8.0g		

Filter list of variables matching any or all keyword(s)

Variable Properties

Name
weikg

Label
weight in kg

Type
byte ▼

Format
%8.0g   Create...

Value label
▼   Manage...

Notes
No notes   Manage...

◄ ►   Reset   Apply

Figure 1.8   Assigning labels to each variable.

To continue working in Stata after having created a database, the user needs to ensure that the data have been saved. To that end, the user will need to assign a name to the file to continue working on the database. Clicking on "File" (on the toolbar) followed by "Save As" (on the subsequent dropdown menu) begins this process. After that, select the working folder or directory and assign a name to the database. The default file extension is .dta.

Chapter 2

Data Description

Aim: Upon completing the chapter, the learner should be able to describe a database with the specific commands of Stata.

2.1 Most Useful Commands

Although specific reference is made to the use of the menus and dialog windows of the program, it is important to understand how to manage the different conditions and options that are available for each Stata command. Most Stata commands follow the same basic sequence:

```
<command> <variable or variables list> <condition or use of
if>, <options>
```

A list containing several of the commands and their corresponding descriptions follows below:

`list`	Lists the values of the variables
`describe`	Produces a summary of the dataset in memory or of the data stored in a Stata-format dataset
`codebook`	Examines the variable names, labels, and data to produce a codebook for describing the dataset
`generate`	Creates a new variable in the dataset
`recode`	Changes the values of the numeric variables according to the rules specified

replace	Changes the contents of an existing variable
label	Can be used for several purposes, but is mainly used for attaching labels to data, variables, or values
drop	Eliminates variables or observations from the data that are in the memory
summarize	Calculates and displays a variety of univariate summary statistics
tabulate	Produces one-way or two-way tables of frequency counts
table	Calculates and displays tables of statistics

2.2 *list* Command

The *list* command displays the values of all the components of the database requested in the command line. If the user wants to view a specific variable of the database, the user must first write the word *list*, followed by the condition *in* and then write the number of observations to be viewed on the screen, as shown in the following:

Output

```
. list in 5/10
       +-------------------------------------+
       | var1    var2    var3    var4    var5 |
       |-------------------------------------|
   5.  |    5      45      56    1.52       1 |
   6.  |    6      36      87    1.46       1 |
   7.  |    7      30      78    1.44       1 |
   8.  |    8      29      77    1.56       1 |
   9.  |    9      27      67    1.52       0 |
       |-------------------------------------|
  10.  |   10      29      63    1.52       1 |
       +-------------------------------------+
```

Only observations 5–10 of the active database are displayed.

2.3 Mathematical and Logical Operators

To carry out different mathematical or logical operations with numbers or variables of the active database, the following symbols are available:

Symbol	Definition
==	Equal to (double equal sign)
!= or ~=	Not equal to
>	Greater than
>=	Greater than or equal to
<	Less than
<=	Less than or equal to
+	Addition (e.g., 2 + 3)
−	Subtraction (e.g., 2 − 3)
*	Multiplication (e.g., 2 * 3)
/	Division (e.g., 2/3)
^	Exponentiation (e.g., 2 ^ 3)
&	*and* (assuming two conditions, the symbol & is used to indicate that both conditions are occurring simultaneously.)
|	*or* (assuming two conditions, the symbol | is used to indicate that one or the other or both conditions are occurring; that is, that at least one of them is occurring.)

Usually, these operators are associated with the conditional command *If* for specific variables. For example, to display only those observations in which the age is below 30, the command line is as follows:

```
list id age weikg heimt if age<30
```

Output

```
      +-------------------------------+
      |  id    age    weikg    heimt  |
      |-------------------------------|
 1.   |   1     28       59     1.55  |
 3.   |   3     25       76      1.6  |
 4.   |   4     26       65     1.78  |
 8.   |   8     29       77     1.56  |
 9.   |   9     27       67     1.52  |
      |-------------------------------|
10.   |  10     29       63     1.52  |
      +-------------------------------+
```

The symbol of asterisk (*) is also used to make any comment during the Stata programming; for example:

```
*Displaying observations in which the age is below 30
list  id age weikg heimt if age<30
```

2.4 *generate* Command

The *generate* command (or *gen*) is used to define new variables in an existing database. For example, let us suppose that you have a database of anthropometric measurements (corresponding to the hypothetical participants of your study), such as weight in kilograms (*weikg*) and height in meters (*heimt*), and you want to calculate the body mass index (*bmi*) of each participant, with bmi being defined as the ratio of weikg over heimt squared. Suppose, further, that the following database is active in Stata:

```
     +-----------------------------------------+
     | id    age    weikg    heimt    sex |
     |-----------------------------------------|
 1.  | 1     28       59     1.55      0  |
 2.  | 2     32       35     1.35      0  |
 3.  | 3     25       76      1.6      0  |
 4.  | 4     26       65     1.78      0  |
 5.  | 5     45       56     1.52      1  |
     |-----------------------------------------|
 6.  | 6     36       87     1.46      1  |
 7.  | 7     30       78     1.44      1  |
 8.  | 8     29       77     1.56      1  |
 9.  | 9     27       67     1.52      0  |
10.  | 10    29       63     1.52      1  |
     +-----------------------------------------+
```

To compute and display the *bmi* of each participant, the following commands are executed:

```
gen bmi = weikg/(heimt^2)
list id bmi
```

You can see that a new variable, named *bmi*, has been created as a result of using the *list* command:

Output

```
      +----------------+
      |  id        bmi |
      |----------------|
  1.  |   1    24.55775 |
  2.  |   2    19.20439 |
  3.  |   3     29.6875 |
  4.  |   4    20.51509 |
  5.  |   5    24.23823 |
      |----------------|
  6.  |   6    40.81441 |
  7.  |   7    37.61574 |
  8.  |   8    31.64037 |
  9.  |   9    28.99931 |
 10.  |  10    27.26801 |
      +----------------+
```

2.5 *recode* Command

The *recode* command allows the user to change or regroup the values of any variable. For example, let us assume that a user wants to regroup the values of the bmi variable of the previous database in the following three groups: (1) Group 1 contains the values ranging from 18.5 to 24.9, (2) Group 2 are those that range from 25 to 29.9, and (3) Group 3 are the values that are 30 or greater. The commands sequence is as follows:

```
gen bmig=bmi
recode bmig 18.5/24.9=1 25/29.9=2 30/max=3
list id bmig
```

Output

```
      +-------------+
      |  id    bmig |
      |-------------|
  1.  |   1       1 |
  2.  |   2       1 |
  3.  |   3       2 |
  4.  |   4       1 |
  5.  |   5       1 |
      |-------------|
  6.  |   6       3 |
  7.  |   7       3 |
  8.  |   8       3 |
  9.  |   9       2 |
 10.  |  10       2 |
      +-------------+
```

2.6 *drop* Command

The *drop* command allows us to eliminate from one to several variables from our active database. For example, to eliminate the bmi variable, the following command must be used:

```
drop bmi
```

2.7 *replace* Command

This command allows you to change the value of an existing variable according to the rule specified. For example, let us assume that a user wants to categorize bmi into the following groups: Group 1 (persons with a bmi from 18.5 to 24.49), Group 2 (persons with a bmi from 24.5 and 29.9), and Group 3 (persons with a bmi from 30 onward). The command sequence to create these categories of bmi, assuming that bmi was not already created, is as follows:

```
gen bmi= weikg/(heimt^2)
gen bmig=bmi
replace bmig=1 if bmi >= 18.5 & bmi < 24.5
replace bmig=2 if bmi >= 24.5 &  bmi < 30
replace bmig=3 if bmi >= 30
list id bmig
```

After the *list* command, the results will be the same as that reported with the *replace* command.

2.8 *label* Command

The *label* command defines a name to the variables of the active database; for example, the *label variable* command assigns a label to the variable bmig as follows:

```
label variable bmig "body mass index categories"
```

In addition, the *label* command decodes the categories of the variables, combining *label define* and *label value* commands. The *label define* command is used to create a label for different codes to be attached to a legend. Then, the *label value* command is used to relate the categories of 1 variable to the labels defined in *label define* command. For example, the command lines that are used to label the codes of the variables sex and *bmig* are as follows:

```
label define sexc 0 "Male" 1 "Female"
label value sex sexc
```

```
label define bm 1 "Normal" 2 "Overweight" 3 "Obese"
label value  bmig bm
list id sex bmig
```

After using the *list* command, the following output will be displayed:

```
    +-----------------------------+
    | id       sex        bmig |
    |-----------------------------|
 1. | 1        Male    Overweight |
 2. | 2        Male       Normal |
 3. | 3        Male    Overweight |
 4. | 4        Male       Normal |
 5. | 5      Female       Normal |
    |-----------------------------|
 6. | 6      Female        Obese |
 7. | 7      Female        Obese |
 8. | 8      Female        Obese |
 9. | 9        Male    Overweight |
10. | 10     Female    Overweight |
    +-----------------------------+
```

If you want to eliminate a label that was previously assigned to a variable, the *drop* command must be used, as follows:

```
label drop sex
```

And to eliminate all of the assigned labels, write the following:

```
label drop all
```

2.9 *summarize* Command

If we want to summarize the variables in a database, we must write *summarize* (or *sum*) in our command window. After we do this, a table containing a summary of all the variables in our database appears. It is recommended that this command be used with quantitative variables. For example, in the previous database, age, weight (*weikg*), height (*heimt*), and bmi are defined as quantitative variables; therefore, the command would be as follows:

```
sum  age weikg heimt bmi
```

Output

Variable	Obs	Mean	Std. Dev.	Min	Max
age	10	30.7	5.9264	25	45
weikg	10	66.3	14.62912	35	87
heimt	10	1.53	.1127435	1.35	1.78
bmi	10	28.45408	6.925241	19.20439	40.81441

As a result, in the command window, a table is displayed containing the number of observations, mean (*Mean*), standard deviation (*Std. Dev.*), minimum (*Min*), and maximum (*Max*) for each variable. If the user is interested in displaying descriptive statistics for certain conditions, the conditional command *if* can be used. For example, a statistical description of the bmi in subjects less than 30 years old, the following procedure can be used:

```
sum bmi if age < 30
```

Output

Variable	Obs	Mean	Std. Dev.	Min	Max
bmi	6	27.11134	4.01918	20.51509	31.64037

The *detail* command can be written at the end of the command line to obtain information, which is more detailed, about quantitative variables in the database. For example, assuming we want the detailed information of the distribution of the variable *bmi,* the following command line can be used:

```
sum bmi, detail
```

Output

bmi

	Percentiles	Smallest		
1%	19.20439	19.20439		
5%	19.20439	20.51509		
10%	19.85974	24.23823	Obs	10
25%	24.23823	24.55775	Sum of Wgt.	10
50%	28.13366		Mean	28.45408
		Largest	Std. Dev.	6.925241
75%	31.64037	29.6875		
90%	39.21507	31.64037	Variance	47.95897
95%	40.81441	37.61574	Skewness	.4458304
99%	40.81441	40.81441	Kurtosis	2.272217

2.10 do-file Editor

A do-file is a set of Stata commands that can be stored for later use. In the Stata toolbar, click on the icon ![icon] to create a do-file. A window will open (Figure 2.1), and you can either type or paste a series of commands and then save this as a file for later use. To execute these commands, totally or partially, click on the *Do* icon, ![icon], in this editor, which is located in the extreme right corner.

Once the sequence of Stata commands is defined for the first time, a name has to be assigned to this do-file for later use. Stata assigns the extension .do to this file name.

2.11 Descriptive Statistics and Graphs

To generate a table of descriptive statistics, on the main taskbar, click **Statistics → Summaries, tables, and tests → Other tables → Compact table of summary statistics** (Figure 2.2).

When you click this sequence, a window opens that lets you select the variable of the active database that will be analyzed and choose the statistical procedure of interest. Within this window, we can assess (in terms of mean, standard deviation, coefficient of variation, 25th percentile [p25], 75th percentile [p75], and interquartile range [p75–p25]) the statistical distribution of a quantitative variable, as shown for *bmi* from the previous database (Figure 2.3).

If the *Statistics* icon is used, Stata displays the command and the results. The output above indicates that the value of the sd (*standard deviation*) is only 24.3% of the mean, which might suggest a relatively moderate variability in the bmi

```
1   gen bmi=weikg/(heimt^2)
2   gen bmig=bmi
3   replace bmig=1 if bmi < 18.5
4   replace bmig=2 if bmi >=18.5 & bmi < 24.9
5   replace bmig=3 if bmi >=24.9 & bmi < 30
6   replace bmig=4 if bmi >=30
7   list id bmig
8
9
```

Figure 2.1 do-file editor window.

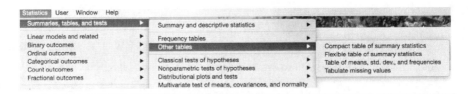

Figure 2.2 Creating a table to display summary statistics.

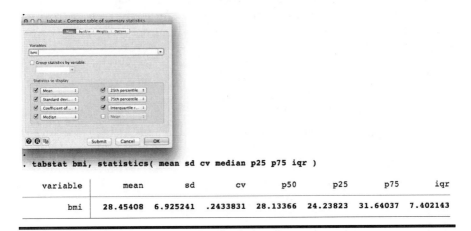

```
. tabstat bmi, statistics( mean sd cv median p25 p75 iqr )
```

variable	mean	sd	cv	p50	p25	p75	iqr
bmi	28.45408	6.925241	.2433831	28.13366	24.23823	31.64037	7.402143

Figure 2.3 Window for displaying a table of summary statistics.

distribution. Based on the iqr (*interquartile range*), the output indicates that 50% of the bmi around the median value is not greater than 7.4.

2.12 *tabulate* Command

The *tabulate* (or *tab*) command provides a table with the frequency values of the corresponding variable. For example, to obtain the frequency distribution of the grouped *bmi* (bmig), the user needs to write the following:

```
tab bmig
```

Output

bmig	Freq.	Percent	Cum.
Normal	3	30.00	30.00
Overweight	4	40.00	70.00
Obese	3	30.00	100.00
Total	10	100.00	

In this example, 30% of the study group was categorized as being obese and 40% as being normal.

The *tab* command can be used to report contingency tables that, in turn, can be used to report the frequency distribution, with the option of including percentages by column and row. For example, to describe the association between the variables *bmig* and *sex* (see the previous database), use the *tab* command, as follows:

```
tab bmig sex, co
```

Output

```
+-------------------+
| Key               |
|-------------------|
|      frequency    |
| column percentage |
+-------------------+

           |        sex
     bmig  |    Male     Female  |    Total
-----------+---------------------+---------
   Normal  |      2          1   |        3
           |  40.00      20.00   |    30.00
-----------+---------------------+---------
Overweight |      3          1   |        4
           |  60.00      20.00   |    40.00
-----------+---------------------+---------
    Obese  |      0          3   |        3
           |   0.00      60.00   |    30.00
-----------+---------------------+---------
    Total  |      5          5   |       10
           | 100.00     100.00   |   100.00
```

The results show that 80% of women are categorized as being either overweight or obese, while 40% of men are categorized as being overweight, with none being categorized as being obese. Only 30% of the subjects (both sexes) are categorized as being of normal weight.

Chapter 3

Graph Construction

Aim: Upon completing the chapter, the learner should be able to create the graphs that are most commonly used for data description.

3.1 Introduction

To create a graph, we click on the *Graphics* option on the taskbar (Figure 3.1). After we do this, the following dropdown menu appears, listing a series of possible graphs that can be constructed.

Afterward, the user clicks the type of graph or plot needed; a new window with the different specifications available for this type of graph will be displayed. Once the specifications are provided, the user must choose one of the following two options for obtaining the graph that he or she desires: *Submit* or *OK*. If *Submit* is chosen, the requested graph will be displayed, with the graph window remaining open (enabling the user to explore other specifications); choosing *OK* brings up the requested graph but the graph window remains closed.

3.2 Box Plot

To construct a box plot, the user should click the *Box Plot* option after clicking *Graphics* (Figure 3.2). Afterward, a quantitative variable must be defined. For example, to obtain the box plot for the variable bmi of the previous database, insert bmi in the space provided; in addition, the user has the option of writing a title in the *Title* option (Figure 3.3).

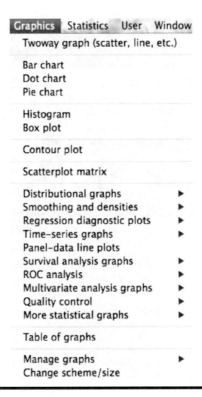

Figure 3.1 Graphics options.

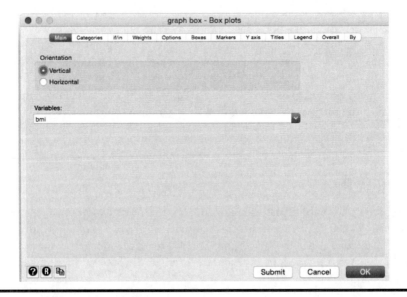

Figure 3.2 Box plot window.

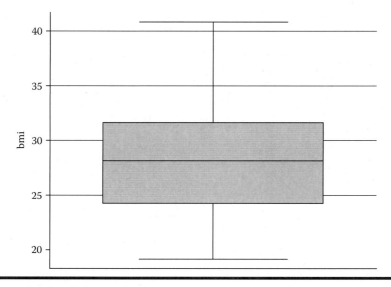

Figure 3.3   Graph box for bmi.

3.3 Histogram

Another commonly used chart is the histogram, which shows the frequency distribution of the variable of interest using abutting rectangles, and in which the height of each rectangle corresponds to the frequency of subjects within certain limits of the variable (these limits are the base of each rectangle). For example, to create a histogram of the variable with four rectangles using the *Graphics* window, the user needs to click the Histogram option and write the name of the variable, bmi (Figure 3.4). At this point, the user has the option of specifying the number of rectangles in the space labeled *Number of bins and*, in addition, has the option to include the normal density plot (see Figure 3.5).

The *normal* option will show a curve of the normal probability distribution over the histogram. This tells us how far away the distribution of the variable of interest is from the normal distribution.

3.4 Bar Chart

To construct a bar chart, the user clicks the *Bar Chart* option after clicking *Graphics* and sets the specifications for this type of graph (Figure 3.6). For example, to show the mean of the bmi by sex, the user needs to define the requested statistics (i.e., mean), and the variable that identifies the subgroup (for the purposes of this example, the variable *sex*) in the window that is opened when the *By* button is depressed (see Figure 3.7).

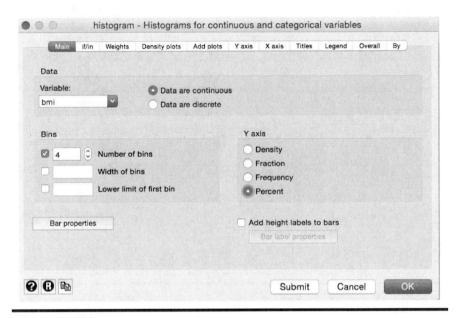

Figure 3.4   Histogram window.

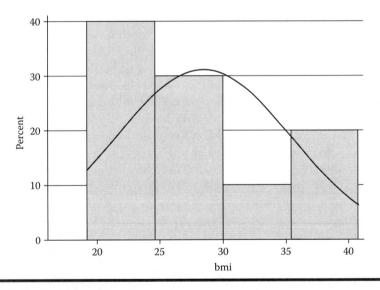

Figure 3.5   Histogram for bmi.

The results show that the mean of the bmi in women is higher than it is in men. The next chapter will demonstrate the procedure that is used to determine whether this sort of difference is statistically significant.

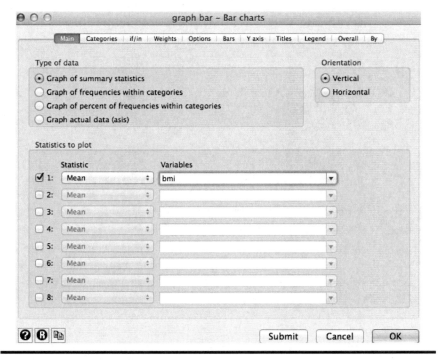

Figure 3.6   Bar chart window.

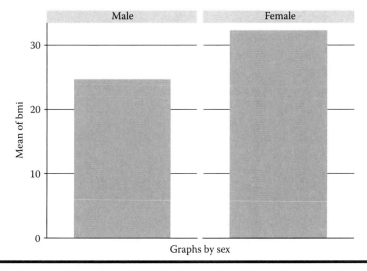

Figure 3.7   Graph bar: Mean bmi by sex.

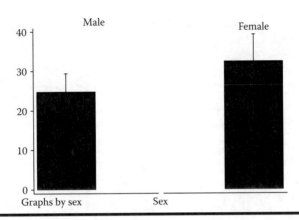

Figure 3.8 Mean bmi with one standard deviation by sex.

Another type of bar chart that the user might want to create is one in which the standard deviation is added (see Figure 3.8). The next sequence of commands can be used for this purpose:

```
sort sex
gen mbmi=bmi
gen sbmi=bmi
collapse (mean) mbmi (sd) sbmi, by(sex)
gen hbmi = mbmi + sbmi
twoway (bar mbmi sex) (rcap hbmi mbmi sex), yscale(range(0 40))
xlabel(none) by(sex, noxrescale) by(,legend(off))
```

The *collapse* command is used to summarize a set of data using statistics, such as mean, sum, median, and percentiles. These statistics can be computed overall or for each category of specific variables, previously sorted. In the last sequence of commands, we computed the mean and standard deviation of the variable bmi for each category of variable sex. The *twoway* command is used to create different plots in the same graph. In the previous example, we used bar for graph bars and rcap for capped spikes in the same graph.

Chapter 4

Significance Tests

Aim: Upon completing the chapter, the learner should be able to perform significance tests that are concerned with the expected values of continuous random variables.

4.1 Introduction

Classical statistical tests are performed to compare the expected values of a random variable, under the assumption that these values are constant parameters of the target population. The Bayesian approach assumes that these parameters are another random variable. In this chapter we will concentrate our analysis using classical statistical tests for comparing the expected values of a continuous random variable in two independent groups.

The classical statistical tests are based on the initial formulation of two complementary hypotheses that are related to the parameters of the target population; these hypotheses are the null and the alternative hypotheses. The null hypothesis, denoted by H_0, is the hypothesis that is to be tested. The alternative hypothesis, usually denoted by H_a, is the hypothesis that contradicts the null hypothesis (Rosner, 2010); usually, the alternative hypothesis will be related to a research hypothesis. To assess the null hypothesis, a sample of data is collected to compute a *test statistic* for supporting a decision in favor of or against the H_0; there are four possible outcomes:

1. Evidence in favor of H_0, with H_0 in fact being true
2. Evidence against H_0, though H_0 is in fact true (Type I error)
3. Evidence in favor of H_0, though H_0 is in fact false (Type II error)
4. Evidence against H_0, with H_0 in fact being false

In classical statistics, the probabilities of the occurrences of these outcomes are summarized in the following table:

Decision based on the sample data	H_0	
	True	*False*
Evidence in favor of H_0 (do not reject H_0)	$1 - \alpha = \Pr[\text{accept } H_0 \mid H_0 \text{ true}]$	$\beta = \Pr[\text{accept } H_0 \mid H_0 \text{ false}]$ *Probability of Type II error*
Evidence against H_0 (reject H_0)	$\alpha = \Pr[\text{reject } H_0 \mid H_0 \text{ true}]$ *Probability of Type I error* **(significance level)**	$1 - \beta = \Pr[\text{reject } H_0 \mid H_0 \text{ false}]$ **Statistical power**

The general aim in hypothesis testing is to use statistical tests that make α and β as small as possible. Typically, the evidence against H_0 is determined with a significance level less than or equal to 5%, while a statistical power of 80% or higher is considered adequate.

The significance level can be defined prior to performing the test; when this is done, two regions for the test statistics are defined: the *acceptance region* (evidence for accepting H_0) and the *rejection region* (evidence against the null hypothesis). However, the output of the statistical programs usually shows the probability (called *P*-value) for each statistical test. *P*-value is defined as the probability of obtaining a test statistic as extreme as or more extreme than the test statistic actually obtained, given that the null hypothesis is true. As a consequence, the *P*-value is interpreted as α level at which the given value of the test statistic is on the borderline between the acceptance and rejection regions (Rosner, 2010). In Stata, the *P*-value will be presented according to the test statistic used and the probability distribution assumed for this statistic; for example, assuming the Student's *t*-test statistic with t-probability distribution, the output for identifying the *P*-value will be expressed as $\Pr(T > t)$. To interpret *P*-values, we can use one of the following statements (Rosner, 2010):

If the *P*-value $\geq .05$, then the results are considered not statistically significant.
If $.01 <$ *P*-value $< .05$, then the results are significant.
If $.001 <$ *P*-value $\leq .01$, then the results are highly significant.
If the *P*-value $\leq .001$, then the results are very highly significant.

However, if $.05 \leq$ *P*-value $< .10$, then a trend toward statistical significance is sometimes noted.

4.2 Normality Test

When we want to estimate or compare the expected value of a continuous random variable, usually we assume that this variable follows a normal probability distribution. To assess whether the normality assumption is met, different statistical tests can be performed. A formal test to evaluate the normality of a continuous random variable is the *Shapiro–Wilk test,* whose null hypothesis states that a given random variable follows a normal distribution (Rosner, 2010). The *swilk* command can be used for this purpose. For example, to determine whether the continuous variables of the previous database follow a normal distribution, the command line below can be used:

```
swilk age weikg heimt bmi
```

Output

```
          Shapiro-Wilk W test for normal data

Variable |    Obs        W         V        z      Prob>z
---------+---------------------------------------------------
     age |     10     0.82089    2.760    1.943    0.02598
   weikg |     10     0.94243    0.887   -0.203    0.58031
   heimt |     10     0.93312    1.031    0.052    0.47923
     bmi |     10     0.95562    0.684   -0.628    0.73506
```

The results above provide evidence in favor of the null hypothesis for all variables (*P*-value > .05) with the exception of the variable age (*P*-value = .0259).

4.3 Variance Homogeneity

An assumption that can be used in the performance of a parametric test to compare the expected values of a continuous random variable in two unmatched groups is that the variances are equal (variance homogeneity). This indicates that the location parameters (expected values) of the continuous random variables can be different in each group, but the dispersion parameter (variance) is equal in all groups. To perform this assessment in two groups, the *sdtest* command is available; for this assessment, it is assumed that the variance ratio of the two groups follows an *F*-Fisher probability distribution $\left(\sigma_1^2 / \sigma_2^2 \sim F \right)$. The command lines are as follows for the variables *bmi, weight,* and *height* (all from the previous database):

```
sdtest  bmi, by(sex)
sdtest  weikg, by(sex)
sdtest  heimt, by(sex)
```

Output

```
. sdtest  bmi, by(sex)

Variance ratio test
------------------------------------------------------------------------
   Group | Obs      Mean   Std. Err. Std. Dev. [95% Conf. Interval]
---------+--------------------------------------------------------------
    Male |   5  24.59281  2.133509  4.770671    18.66924    30.51638
  Female |   5  32.31535  3.094344  6.919164    23.72407    40.90663
---------+--------------------------------------------------------------
combined |  10  28.45408  2.189954  6.925241    23.50006     33.4081
------------------------------------------------------------------------
     ratio = sd(Male) / sd(Female)                         f = 0.4754
Ho: ratio = 1                            degrees of freedom =   4, 4

   Ha: ratio < 1            Ha: ratio != 1             Ha: ratio > 1
 Pr(F < f) = 0.2446    2*Pr(F < f) = 0.4891       Pr(F > f) = 0.7554

. sdtest  weik, by(sex)

Variance ratio test
------------------------------------------------------------------------
   Group | Obs    Mean   Std. Err.  Std. Dev.  [95% Conf. Interval]
---------+--------------------------------------------------------------
    Male |   5   60.4   6.910861   15.45316    41.21237    79.58763
  Female |   5   72.2   5.580323   12.47798    56.70654    87.69346
---------+--------------------------------------------------------------
combined |  10   66.3   4.626133   14.62912    55.83496    76.76504
------------------------------------------------------------------------
     ratio = sd(Male) / sd(Female)                         f = 1.5337
Ho: ratio = 1                            degrees of freedom =   4, 4

   Ha: ratio < 1            Ha: ratio != 1             Ha: ratio > 1
 Pr(F < f) = 0.6556    2*Pr(F > f) = 0.6887       Pr(F > f) = 0.3444

. sdtest  heimt, by(sex)

Variance ratio test
------------------------------------------------------------------------
   Group | Obs   Mean   Std. Err.  Std. Dev.  [95% Conf. Interval]
---------+--------------------------------------------------------------
    Male |   5   1.56   .0692098   .1547579    1.367843    1.752157
  Female |   5    1.5   .0219089   .0489897    1.439171    1.560829
---------+--------------------------------------------------------------
combined |  10   1.53   .0356526   .1127435    1.449348    1.610652
------------------------------------------------------------------------
     ratio = sd(Male) / sd(Female)                         f = 9.9792
Ho: ratio = 1                            degrees of freedom =   4, 4

   Ha: ratio < 1            Ha: ratio != 1             Ha: ratio > 1
 Pr(F < f) = 0.9766    2*Pr(F > f) = 0.0468       Pr(F > f) = 0.0234
```

For each variable (in the above case, *sex*), a table displays a description of the summary measures in each category of that variable: *Obs* (number of observations), *Mean, Std. Err.* (standard error), *Std. Dev.* (standard deviation), and 95% Conf. Interval (the 95% confidence interval is used to estimate the expected value of the random variables). In the above table, the user can see that the standard deviation of the variable bmi among males is 4.77 (variance = 22.75), while among females it is 6.92 (variance = 47.74); so the estimated ratio of the variances is 0.4754 (male/female). If the variances are equal in these two groups, the expected value of this ratio must be 1 (Rosner, 2010). Near the bottom of the table, the user can see that the null hypothesis is "H_0: ratio = 1." The alternative hypothesis is expressed in three ways: H_a: ratio < 1, H_a: ratio != 1 (different than 1), and H_a: ratio > 1; it is recommended that only the second alternative hypothesis *(ratio is different from 1)* be considered, if the purpose is assessing the variance homogeneity. Below each alternative hypothesis, the corresponding *P*-values are presented. Only for the variable *height* does the statistical evidence not support the assumption of variance homogeneity (*P*-value = .0468).

4.4 Student's *t*-Test for Independent Samples

Assuming that the assumptions of normality and variance homogeneity are met, the next step is to determine whether the expected value of the continuous variable changes in different groups. Suppose that the user wants to compare the expected value of the variable bmi by sex, assuming that the selection of a male is independent of the selection of a female in the study sample; for this, Student's *t*-test for independent samples (Rosner, 2010) can be used, as is demonstrated with the following expression:

$$t = \frac{\bar{Y}_1 - \bar{Y}_2}{\sqrt{\mathrm{Var}\left(\bar{Y}_1 - \bar{Y}_2\right)}} \sim t_{k|H_0}$$

where:
$\bar{Y}_i$ indicates the sample mean of the variable bmi for the *i*th group
t_k is the *t-probability distribution* with k degrees of freedom
$\mathrm{Var}\left(\bar{Y}_1 - \bar{Y}_2\right)$ is the variance of $\left(\bar{Y}_1 - \bar{Y}_2\right)$

To compute the *P*-value, it is assumed that this expression follows the *t-probability distribution* under the null hypothesis assumption. To perform this kind of *t*-test, the user can utilize the *ttest* command. The specifications for this command can change depending on the structure of the database. For example, assuming that the previous database is being used and that the aim of the user is to assess the variance homogeneity in the variable bmi by sex group, the command line for performing student's *t*-test is as follows:

```
ttest bmi, by(sex)
```

Output

Two-sample t test with equal variances

Group	Obs	Mean	Std. Err.	Std. Dev.	[95% Conf. Interval]	
"Male"	5	24.59281	2.133509	4.770671	18.66924	30.51638
"Female"	5	32.31535	3.094344	6.919164	23.72407	40.90663
combined	10	28.45408	2.189954	6.925241	23.50006	33.4081
diff		-7.722543	3.758567		-16.38981	.9447286

```
    diff = mean("Male") - mean("Female")              t = -2.0547
Ho: diff = 0                        degrees of freedom =        8

    Ha: diff < 0          Ha: diff != 0               Ha: diff > 0
Pr(T < t) = 0.0370   Pr(|T| > |t|) = 0.0740    Pr(T > t) =   0.9630
```

The above table is the same as the one described by the *sdtest* command. However, the null hypothesis formulated below in this table is different. The null hypothesis states that the expected bmi value is the same for both sexes $(\mu_{Male} = \mu_{Female})$. In Stata notation, this hypothesis is formulated as the following: diff = mean(Male) − mean(Fem) = 0. The alternative hypotheses that can be assessed are H_a: diff < 0, H_a: diff != 0 *(different than zero)*, and H_a: diff > 0. Assuming that the research hypothesis is that *males have a lower mean body mass index than females do,* the user has to assess the *P*-value below the first alternative hypothesis (one-tailed alternative hypothesis), with the result indicating that there is statistical evidence against the null hypothesis (*P*-value = .037); this finding suggests that the expected bmi in males is lower than the expected bmi in females. If the research hypothesis is that *males have different mean body mass index than females do,* then the user has to assess the *P*-value below the second alternative hypothesis (two-tailed alternative hypothesis), with this result indicating that there is statistical evidence in favor of the null hypothesis (*P*-value = .074); this finding suggests that the expected bmi in males is not different from the expected bmi in females.

4.5 Confidence Intervals for Testing the Null Hypothesis

Another way to assess the null hypothesis is to use a confidence interval. For example, to assess the statistical hypotheses, the following can be used: $H_0 : \mu_{Male} - \mu_{Female} = 0$ vs. $H_a : \mu_{Male} - \mu_{Female} \neq 0$. In this case, to test the null hypothesis (with a 5% significance level), the 95% confidence level for the mean difference provided in the *ttest* command can be used. The interval indicates that with a 95% confidence level, the difference of the expected bmi by sex $(\mu_{Male} - \mu_{Female})$ is between -16.39 and 0.94. As zero is included in the interval, this finding provides evidence in favor of the null hypothesis (P-value $> .05$).

4.6 Nonparametric Tests for Unpaired Groups

There are several tests available to assess the distribution of the quantitative random variable in two groups when the basic assumptions of the *t*-test are violated. One of these tests is the *Mann–Whitney test,* also called the *Wilcoxon rank sum test,* which is a nonparametric test that compares two unpaired groups. To perform the Mann–Whitney test, all data are ranked, paying no attention to which group each value belongs; the smallest number gets a rank of 1 and the largest number gets a rank of n, where n is the total number of values in the two groups. Then, this test computes the average of the ranks in each group and reports the two averages. If the means of the ranks in the two groups are very different, the P-value will be small. The null hypothesis is that the distributions of both groups will be identical, so that there is a 50% probability that an observation from a value randomly selected from one population will exceed an observation randomly selected from the other population. In Stata, this test can be performed with the command *kwallis*. Using the data from the previous example, the syntax of the *kwallis* command is as follows:

```
kwallis bmi, by(sex)
```

Output

```
Kruskal-Wallis equality-of-populations rank test
+----------------------------+
|    sex | Obs | Rank Sum |
|--------+-----+----------|
|   Male |  5  |   20.00  |
| Female |  5  |   35.00  |
+----------------------------+
```

```
chi-squared =        2.455 with 1 d.f.
probability =        0.1172

chi-squared with ties =       2.455 with 1 d.f.
probability =        0.1172
```

As can be seen above, the results of this test show that the frequency distributions of the bmi for both sexes are identical (*P*-value = .1172). This interpretation is consistent with that of Student's *t*-test for the two-tailed alternative hypothesis. An extensive review of the parametric and nonparametric statistical procedures can be found in the book of Sheskin (2007).

4.7 Sample Size and Statistical Power

The study design for comparing two means involves the minimum sample size and statistical power needed to reduce the probability of a false conclusion. Stata provides the *Power and sample size* option on the *Statistics* dropdown menu (Figure 4.1).

Once the *Statistics* menu is clicked, a new window will be displayed (Figure 4.2). If you choose the test comparing two independent means, a dialog window, in which the user enters the data according to the study problem, is displayed. For example, assuming that we are interested in determining the minimum sample size of the previous example for a two-sided test with a 5% significance level, an 80% statistical power, and an allocation ratio equal to 1 (equal sample size in each group), the window should be completed in the manner seen in Figure 4.3.

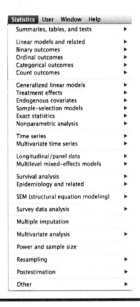

Figure 4.1   Statistics options.

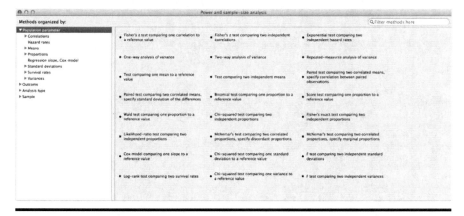

Figure 4.2   Power and sample size analysis options.

power twomeans – Power analysis for a two-sample means test

Main | Table | Graph | Iteration

Compute: * Accepts numlist (Examples)

Total sample size   ⇕

Error probabilities

0.05   * Significance level   0.8   * Power   ⇕

Sample size

1   * Allocation ratio, N2/N1
☐ Allow fractional sample sizes

Effect size

Means   Standard deviations

24.6   * Control   ○ Common standard deviation
32.2   * Experimental ⇕   1   * Common value
                                         ⊙ Group standard deviations
                                            4.77   * Control
                                            6.91   * Experimental
                                         ☐ Assume a known standard deviations

Sides:

Two-sided test ⇕

Figure 4.3   Power analyses for a two-sample means test.

After clicking the *Submit* option, the output will be as seen below:

```
. power twomeans 24.6 32.3, sd1(4.77) sd2(6.91)

Performing iteration ...

Estimated sample sizes for a two-sample means test
Satterthwaite's t test assuming unequal variances
Ho: m2 = m1   versus   Ha: m2 != m1

Study parameters:

        alpha =     0.0500
        power =     0.8000
        delta =     7.7000
           m1 =    24.6000
           m2 =    32.3000
          sd1 =     4.7700
          sd2 =     6.9100

Estimated sample sizes:

            N =        22
  N per group =        11
```

To compare the statistical hypotheses with a 5% significance level, an 80% statistical power, and an allocation ratio equal to 1, the minimum sample size needed (for this problem) is 11 per group. If the user is interested in displaying a graph for different options in the statistical power (0.8, 0.85, 0.9), using common standard deviation (5), and different allocation ratios (1, 2, 3), the window should be completed in the manner seen in Figure 4.4.

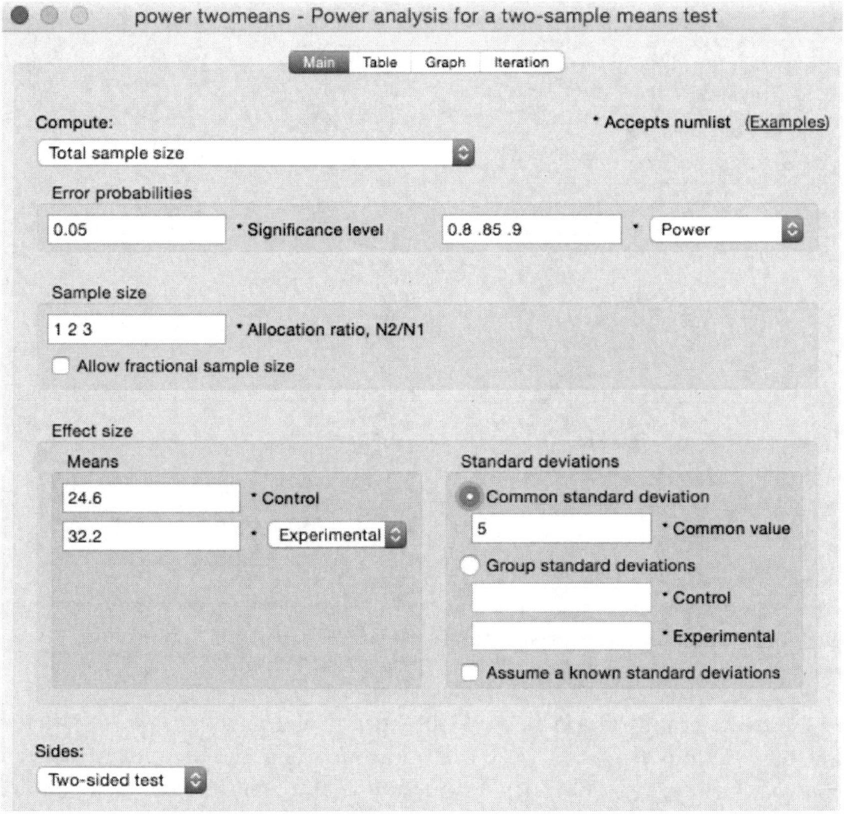

Figure 4.4 Sample size for two-sample means tests with several power levels and allocation ratios.

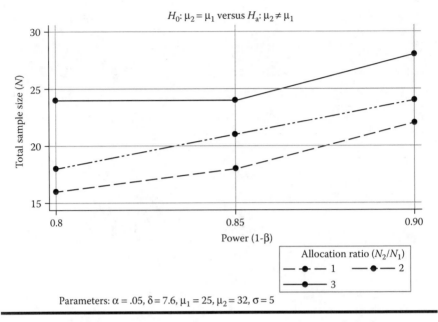

Figure 4.5 Sample size for two-sample means tests using graph option.

When the graph option is used, the output will be as seen in Figure 4.5. The total sample size requested will increase when the statistical power is increased; however, the changes in the sample size will depend on the allocation ratio.

Chapter 5

Linear Regression Models

Aim: Upon completing the chapter, the learner should be able to use *simple, multiple,* and *polynomial linear regression models* for estimating the expected values of a continuous random variable.

5.1 Introduction

A simple linear regression model (SLRM) is a statistical technique that attempts to model the relationship between two variables. One of these variables is the main outcome of interest and is a quantitative random variable, usually denoted with the letter Y and called the *response* or *dependent* variable. The second one can also be quantitative and is used to explain the behavior of the expected values of Y; it is usually denoted with the letter X and is called the *predictor, explanatory,* or *independent* variable. The relationship between these variables, when X is a quantitative variable, is established using the following expression:

$$\mu_{y_i|x_i} = \beta_0 + \beta_1 * x_i$$

where:

$\mu_{y_i|x_i}$ defines the expected value of the random variable Y given the predictor variable X for the ith subject

β_1 is a constant parameter associated with the predictor variable X; it is known as the *slope* of the regression line and indicates the change in the expected value of Y per unit of change in X

β_0 is a constant parameter that indicates the expected value of Y when $x_i = 0$; it is known as the *intercept* of the regression line

A simple regression model can also be expressed with the following formula:

$$y_i = \beta_0 + \beta_1 X_i + e_i$$

where:

y_i indicates the response or dependent variables for the ith subject

e_i denotes the *residual*, which is the difference between the observed values in Y_i and the expected value under the model $\beta_0 + \beta_1 * x_i$ for the ith subject, as follows:

$$e_i = (y_i - \beta_0 + \beta_1 * x_i)$$

5.2 Model Assumptions

The procedure to estimate the regression coefficients of an SLRM is performed based on the following assumptions:

1. The response variable is a quantitative random variable that follows a normal distribution with an expected value of $\beta_0 + \beta_1 * x_i$ and a variance of $\sigma_{Y|X}^2$.

$$Y \sim N\left(\beta_0 + \beta_1 * x_i, \sigma_{Y|X}^2\right)$$

The expected value of the random variable Y is a straight-line function of X.

2. There is independence between the response variable values.

3. The independent or predictor variable is a quantitative variable, not necessarily a random one.

4. The β_i coefficients should not be affected by any power, other than the unit, or by any trigonometric function.

5. The expected value of the residuals is zero, that is,

$$E(e_i) = 0 \quad \text{for every value of "}i\text{"}$$

6. The variance of the residuals is constant and is equal to the variance of the response variable under the SLRM, that is,

$$\mathrm{var}(e_i) = \sigma_{Y/X}^2$$

This variance is constant across the range of values of X (*Homoscedasticity* property).

7. There is no correlation between the residuals, in that

$$E(e_i, e_j) = 0 \quad \text{for all, } i \neq j$$

The residual associated with a subject does not affect the residual of another subject.

8. The probability distribution of the residuals is normal, as can be determined using the following:

$$e_i \sim N\left(0, \sigma_{Y/X}^2\right)$$

5.3 Parameter Estimation

Several methods are available for estimating the beta coefficients for the linear regression model. In classical statistics, the method of *least squares* is used. This method chooses the coefficients that minimize the following residual sum of squares:

$$S = \sum_{i=1}^{n}\left(y_i - \hat{y}_i\right)^2$$

where:

y_i indicates the observed value of the y variable for the ith subject
$\hat{y}_i$ indicates the estimated expected value of Y under the model for the ith subject using a specific combination of the estimated beta coefficients, as follows:

$$\hat{y}_i = \hat{\beta}_0 + \hat{\beta}_1 X_i$$

To reach the coefficients that minimize S, the mathematical method of optimization is used, which equates the first derivative of S to 0 (Draper and Smith, 1998). As a consequence, the resulting equation $\left(\hat{\beta}_0 + \hat{\beta}_1 X_i\right)$ minimizes the distance between the fitted values ($\hat{y}_i$) and the observed values (y_i).

5.4 Hypothesis Testing

To assess the statistical significance of the changes in the expected value of Y per unit of change in X, any one of several methods can be used (Bingham and Fry, 2010). The null hypothesis of these methods states that the coefficient associated with the predictor variable is zero (H_0: $\beta_1 = 0$). One of the methods for testing this hypothesis is the t-test, which is expressed in the following way:

$$t = \frac{\hat{\beta}_1}{\sqrt{\text{Var}\left(\hat{\beta}_1\right)}} \sim t_{n-2|H_0}$$

in which $\hat{\beta}_1$ indicates the estimated β_1, t_{n-2} is the *t-probability distribution* with $n - 2$ degrees of freedom under the null hypothesis, and $\text{Var}\left(\hat{\beta}_1\right)$ is the variance of β_1. To compute the P-value, it is assumed that this formula follows the t-probability distribution under the null hypothesis assumption.

Another method is called *analysis of variance* (ANOVA), which decomposes the variance of Y, as follows:

$$\text{TSS} = \text{SSR} + \text{SSE}$$

where:

$\text{TSS} = \sum_{i=1}^{n}(y_i - \bar{y})^2$ indicates the variation of Y around the overall mean of Y; this variation is known as the *total sum of squares*

$\text{SSR} = \sum_{i=1}^{n}(\hat{y}_i - \bar{y})^2$ indicates the variation due to the *model*, the explained variation between the expected value under the model and the overall mean of Y; this variation is known as *the sum of squares* (SS) due to the regression model

$\text{SSE} = \sum_{i=1}^{n}(y_i - \hat{y})^2$ indicates the overall variation *within* the model and the unexplained variation within the residuals; this variation is known as the *residual sum of squares* or *error sum of squares*

SS divided by their degrees of freedom are the *mean squares* (MS). The following ANOVA table summarizes the sources of variation in the data, SS due to the source, degrees of freedom in the source, MS due to the source, and the expected value of the MS (Draper and Smith, 1998):

Source of Variation	Sum of Squares (SS)	Degrees of Freedom (df)	Mean Squares (MS = SS/df)	Expected Value of MS
Regression	SSR	1	SSR/1	$\sigma^2 + \beta_1^2 \sum_{i=1}^{n}(X_i - \bar{X})^2$
Residual (error)	SSE	$n - 2$	SSE/$(n - 2)$	σ^2
Total	TSS	$n - 1$		

Under the null hypotheses, the ratio $\left\{\left[\sigma^2 + \beta_1^2 \sum(X_i - \bar{X})^2\right]/\sigma^2\right\} = 1$. To determine how far this ratio should be away from 1, once a set data are collected and the parameters of the linear model (σ^2, β_i) are estimated, a P-value is computed using the F-Fisher probability distribution with 1 and $n - 2$ degrees of freedom.

5.5 Coefficient of Determination

The coefficient of determination R^2 is a measure of the goodness of fit of the model and is defined using the following expression:

$$R^2 = \frac{\text{SSR}}{\text{TSS}} \times 100\%$$

where the range of values of R^2 is between 0% and 100%. This coefficient determines the percentage of variation of the variable Y explained by the model. Another way to calculate R^2 is with the following formula:

$$R^2 = 1 - \frac{\text{SSE}}{\text{TSS}} \times 100\%$$

This coefficient is used as a criterion to compare two or more models; the higher the R^2, the better the model fits the data.

5.6 Pearson Correlation Coefficient

The Pearson correlation coefficient is an index indicating the direction and strength of the linear association between two continuous random variables. This coefficient is represented by ρ; the estimator is represented by $r = \hat{\rho}$. Its values range from –1.0 to 1.0. If r is close to 1.0 or to –1.0, it is said that there is a strong positive (directly proportional) or negative (inversely proportional) linear association, respectively; values close to zero indicate little or no linear association. The mathematical expression of r is the following:

$$r = \frac{\text{SSXY}}{\sqrt{\text{SSX} * \text{TSS}}}$$

where:

$$\text{SSXY} = \sum_{i=1}^{n} \left(X_i - \bar{X} \right) \left(Y_i - \bar{Y} \right)$$

and

$$\text{SSX} = \sum_{i=1}^{n} \left(X_i - \bar{X} \right)^2$$

An alternative way to calculate the Pearson correlation coefficient is using the square root of the coefficient of determination, assigning the sign of the β_1 previously estimated:

$$r = \text{sign}\left(\hat{\beta}_1 \right) \sqrt{R^2}$$

To assess whether the Pearson correlation coefficient is different from zero (H_0: $\rho = 0$), with data from a random sample of size n, the following formula is used (Kleinbaum et al., 2008):

$$T = \frac{r\sqrt{n-2}}{\sqrt{1-r^2}} \sim t_{n-2}$$

To obtain the *P*-value, the *t-distribution* with $n - 2$ degrees of freedom is used. This test is equivalent to the *t*-test for assessing H_0: $\beta_1 = 0$, described previously.

5.7 Scatter Plot

Prior to performing a linear regression analysis for specific data, it is recommended that a scatter plot of the observed data be done to determine whether a linear trend can be associated with the relationship that exists between the dependent and independent variables. For example, the relationship between the variables *weight* and *height* (from the previous database) can be obtained (Figure 5.1) with the following command:

```
twoway (scatter weikg heimt) (lfit weikg heimt),
xtitle("Height, mt") ytitle("Weight, kg")
```

Output

The option *lfit* in the *twoway* command is used to draw a line to describe the linear relationship between two variables using an SLRM: in this case between *height* and *weight* given the observed data.

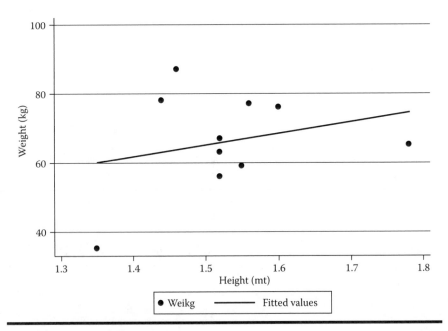

Figure 5.1   Scatter plot.

5.8 Running the Model

The results of this scatter plot show a linear upward trend between height and weight. Specifically, the higher the subjects, the heavier their weight. After generating a scatter plot, the user can run a linear regression model with these data using the command *regress* (or *reg*), as follows:

```
reg weikg heimt
```

Output

```
  Source|     SS        df      MS          Number of obs  =        10
--------+-----------------------------       F(1, 8)        =      0.56
   Model| 125.560422    1   125.560422       Prob > F       =    0.4765
Residual| 1800.53958    8   225.067447       R-squared      =    0.0652
--------+-----------------------------       Adj R-squared  =   -0.0517
   Total|    1926.1     9   214.011111       Root MSE       =    15.002

------------------------------------------------------------------------
   weikg|   Coef.    Std. Err.    t     P>|t|    [95% Conf. Interval]
--------+---------------------------------------------------------------
   heimt| 33.12939   44.35508   0.75   0.476    -69.15362      135.4124
   _cons| 15.61203   68.0289    0.23   0.824    -141.2629      172.487
------------------------------------------------------------------------
```

The results of this command show two tables. The first table describes the estimated ratio of the MS obtained by the model over the residual MS is less than 1 $\left[(125.6/225.1) = 0.56\right]$. This result indicates that there is no evidence to reject the null hypothesis (*P*-value = .4765 > .05). The second table shows the estimated coefficients of the model for the predictor weight and for the intercept (_cons); so, the linear trend is estimated using the following equation: Weight = 15.6 + 33.1 * height. Thus, the estimated expected weight in kilograms will increase 33.1 (95% CI: –69.2, 135.4) for every additional meter of height. However, this increasing trend was not significant (*P*-value > .05). The percentage of total variation from $\bar{Y}$ explained by the model is 6.5% (*R*-squared). In this case, Student's *t*-test described below the ANOVA table shows nonsignificant results for the predictor *weight* with exactly the same *P*-value described for the *F*-distribution in ANOVA, which is because of the fact that in an SLRM, $t^2 = F$.

5.9 Centering

To facilitate the interpretation of the intercept on a linear regression model, it is advisable to transform the values of X_i to the difference of each value from its mean as $\left(X_i - \bar{X}_i\right)$. This transformation is known as *centering*. As a result of the centralization, the estimator of the coefficient associated with the intercept is equal to the mean of the dependent variable, that is,

$$\hat{\beta}_0 = \bar{Y}$$

This process does not affect the estimates of the coefficients associated with the independent variable. Assuming the previous database, the process of centering height to explain weight in STATA can be achieved by typing the following commands:

```
sum weikg
sum heimt
*Centering weikg using the result of the previous sum command
gen heimtc=heimt-r(mean)
reg weikg heimtc
```

Output

```
sum weikg
    Variable  |      Obs      Mean     Std. Dev.    Min        Max
--------------+----------------------------------------------------
       weikg  |       10      66.3     14.62912     35          87

  .          sum heimt

    Variable  |      Obs      Mean     Std. Dev.    Min        Max
--------------+----------------------------------------------------
       heimt  |       10      1.53     .1127435    1.35       1.78
```

```
*Centering weikg using the result of the previous sum command
gen heimtc=heimt-r(mean)
```

```
reg weikg heimtc
    Source  |     SS        df       MS         Number of obs  =       10
------------+------------------------------     F(1, 8)        =     0.56
     Model  | 125.56044     1    125.56044      Prob > F       =   0.4765
  Residual  |1800.53956     8   225.067445      R-squared      =   0.0652
------------+------------------------------     Adj R-squared  =  -0.0517
     Total  |   1926.1      9   214.011111      Root MSE       =   15.002

---------------------------------------------------------------------------
     weikg  |    Coef.    Std. Err.     t     P>|t|    [95% Conf. Interval]
------------+--------------------------------------------------------------
    heimtc  | 33.12939   44.35508     0.75    0.476   -69.15361 135.4124
     _cons  |    66.3     4.744127    13.98    0.000    55.36002 77.23998
---------------------------------------------------------------------------
```

Now the equation model can be expressed in the following manner:

$$\widehat{\text{weikg}} = 66.3 + 33.1 * \text{heimtc} = 66.3 + 33.1 * (\text{heimt} - 1.53)$$

where $\widehat{weikg}$ is the estimated expected weight (kilograms), explained by centering height (meters). The user can confirm that the output is the same with the exception of the estimated constant coefficient ($\hat{\beta}_0 = 66.3$), which is the mean of the variable *weight* and is identified in Stata in the row labeled *_cons*.

5.10 Bootstrapping

Bootstrapping is a robust alternative to classical statistical methods when the assumptions are not met using these methods; it provides more accurate inferences, particularly when the sample size is small. The procedure to perform bootstrapping is via resampling methods for estimating standard errors and computing confidence intervals (Good, 2006). Bootstrapping in Stata can be done using the option *vce(boot)* in the command *reg*. For example, assuming the previous database, the command for estimating weight with centering height using bootstrapping estimates is as follows:

```
reg weikg heimtc, vce(boot)
```

Output

```
Bootstrap replications (50)
----+--- 1 ---+--- 2 ---+--- 3 ---+--- 4 ---+--- 5
..................................................    50

Linear regression                 Number of obs    =          10
                                  Replications     =          50
                                  Wald chi2(1)     =        0.24
                                  Prob > chi2      =      0.6275
                                  R-squared        =      0.0652
                                  Adj R-squared    =     -0.0517
                                  Root MSE         =     15.0022
```

	Observed Coef.	Bootstrap Std. Err.	z	P>|z|	[95% Conf. Interval]	
weikg						
heimtc	33.12939	68.2667	0.49	0.627	-100.6709	166.9297
_cons	66.3	4.538575	14.61	0.000	57.40456	75.19544

The results show that the estimates of the regression coefficients are the same as those obtained using the least-squares method, but the standard errors for the coefficient of heimtc are different, being 44.4 versus 68.3. It is likely that these differences are due to the small sample size that was used in this example. For more information on this topic, we recommend checking out the book by Draper and Smith (1998).

5.11 Multiple Linear Regression Model

An extension of the SLRM is to use more predictor variables to improve the estimation of the expected value of Y. This model extension is called a multiple linear regression model (MLRM), and it is represented as follows for m-predictors:

$$\mu_{y/x} = \beta_0 + \beta_1 X_1 + \cdots + \beta_m X_m$$

where:

$\mu_{y/x}$ indicates the expected value of Y explained by the X variables for the ith subject

X_j indicates the predictor variables ($j = 1,\ldots, m$)

β_j indicates the coefficient (constant) associated with X_j

The assessment of the overall significance of its regression coefficients (β_is, $i > 0$) can be performed using an ANOVA table, as follows:

Source of Variation	SS	df	MS	F-Ratio
Regression	SSR	m	MSR = SSR/m	F_c = MSR/MSE
Residual	SSE	$n - m - 1$	MSE = SSE/($n - m - 1$)	
Total	TSS	$n - 1$	MST = TSS/($n - 1$)	

$$\text{TSS} = \sum_{i=1}^{n} \left(y_i - \bar{y} \right)^2$$

$$\text{SSR} = \sum_{i=1}^{n} \left(\hat{y}_i - \bar{y} \right)^2$$

$$\text{SSE} = \sum_{i=1}^{n} \left(y_i - \hat{y}_i \right)^2$$

where:

$\hat{y}_i$ indicates the estimated expected value of Y given a set of specific values of the predictors

Xs for the ith subject, as follows: $\hat{y}_i = \hat{\beta}_0 + \hat{\beta}_1 X_1 + \ldots + \hat{\beta}_m X_m$

$\hat{\beta}_j$ indicates the estimated value of the coefficient β_j

$\bar{y}_i$ indicates the overall mean of Y

For a multiple regression model, the ANOVA table assumes that H_0: $\beta_1 = \beta_2 = \ldots = \beta_m = 0$. If the calculated value of the test statistic F_c is greater than $F_{(1-\alpha;\ m,\ n-m-1)}$ for a given significance level α, we conclude that there is evidence against H_0.

In MLRMs, the Stata command *reg* can be used in a manner that is similar to how the simple linear regression was programmed, except that in the latter, the model consists of more than one independent variable. For example, assuming the previous database, to explain the expected *bmi* by the predictors *age* and *sex*, the specifications of the *reg* command are as follows:

```
reg  bmi age sex
```

Output

```
   Source |       SS       df   MS              Number of obs  =       10
----------+------------------------------       F( 2,      7)  =     2.81
    Model | 192.330078    2 96.1650389          Prob > F       =  0.1269
 Residual | 239.30065     7 34.1858072          R-squared      =  0.4456
----------+------------------------------       Adj R-squared  =  0.2872
    Total | 431.630728    9 47.9589698          Root MSE       =  5.8469
------------------------------------------------------------------------------
      bmi |     Coef.   Std.Err.     t    P>|t|   [95% Conf. Interval]
----------+-------------------------------------------------------------------
      age | -.4433135  .3941954   -1.12  0.298  -1.375438    .4888106
      sex |  10.47109  4.432552    2.36  0.050  -.0102331    20.95241
    _cons |  36.82826  11.1896     3.29  0.013   10.36907    63.28745
------------------------------------------------------------------------------
```

The results show that the fitted MLRM is

$$\widehat{\text{bmi}} = 36.83 - 0.44 * \text{age} + 10.47 * \text{sex}$$

with *adjusted* $\hat{R}^2 = 28.72\%$. The overall assessment of ANOVA indicates that we are unable to reject the null hypothesis ($H_0: \beta_{\text{age}} = \beta_{\text{sex}} = 0$); thus, this result suggests that the coefficients of the predictors are equal to zero (*P*-value > .05), but the *t*-test for the predictor *sex* suggests that its coefficient in the model could be different from zero (*P*-value = .05). This contradictory result could be explained by the linear dependency (or *multicollinearity*) between the predictors, which affects the procedure that is used to estimate the coefficients of the MLRM. For example, if we want to run the SLRM of each predictor, bmi explained by age and bmi explained by sex, the resulting equations are as follows:

$$\widehat{bmi} = 26.30 + 0.07 * age$$

and

$$\widehat{bmi} = 24.59 + 7.72 * sex$$

When we compare the coefficient estimates of these equations with the equation of the MLRM, we can see different estimates in the coefficient values: 0.07 vs. –0.44 in *age* and 7.72 vs. 10.47 in *sex*. The presence of one of them affects the estimate of the coefficient associated with the other predictor. Unless both predictors are completely independent of each other, the coefficient estimates will not be affected by the presence or absence of one of them (Draper and Smith, 1998).

5.12 Partial Hypothesis

When ANOVA results are significant in MLRMs, the user may wish to determine which set of specific predictor variables are the most significant when all the predictors are assessed simultaneously. For this evaluation, it is recommended that the additional sum of squares of the residuals in the model without these predictors (*incomplete model*) be compared, using the model with these predictors (*complete model*) as a reference. When we reduce the predictor variables from a linear regression model, the sum of squares of the residuals increases. For example, the residual sum of squares for bmi explained by different predictors is described in the following table:

Predictors in the Model	Residual Degrees of Freedom	Residual Sum of Squares	Additional Sum of Squares
Age + sex (complete model)	7	239.3	–
Age (incomplete model)	8	430.1	190.8
Sex (incomplete model)	8	282.5	43.2

In both incomplete models, the additional sum of squares increases. To assess if this increment is statistically significant, a partial F-statistic is used. For example, let us assume the following notation for the complete and incomplete models:

Complete Model: $\mu_{y|X} = \beta_0 + \beta_1 X_1 + \dots + \beta_k X_k + \beta_{k+1} X_{k+1} + \dots + \beta_m X_m$

Nested or Incomplete Model: $\mu_{y|X'} = \beta'_0 + \beta'_1 X_1 + \dots + \beta'_k X_k$

The user has to be aware that the coefficients from both models do not necessarily have the same value. Based on these models, a partial hypothesis can be defined with the following equation:

$$H_0 : \beta_{k+1} = \beta_{k+2} = \ldots = \beta_m = 0 \big|_{X_1, X_2, \ldots, X_k}$$

Then, the following steps are performed to evaluate this type of partial hypothesis:

1. Calculate the sum of squares of the residuals in the complete model (SSE_{com}) with $n - m - 1$ degrees of freedom.
2. Calculate the sum of squares of the residuals in the incomplete model (SSE_{inc}) with $n - k - 1$ degrees of freedom.
3. Compute the difference of SS between the sum of squares of the complete and incomplete models, which is called the additional sum of squares, with $m - k$ degrees of freedom.
4. Compute the following formula (partial F):

$$F\left(X_{k+1}, \ldots, X_m \middle| X_1, \ldots, X_k\right) = \frac{\left(\text{SSE}_{inc} - \text{SSE}_{com}\right)/\left(m - k\right)}{\text{SSE}_{com}/\left(n - m - 1\right)}$$

5. Calculate the P-value using Fisher's F-distribution with $m - k$ and $n - m - 1$ degrees of freedom.

Considering the previous data of the sum of squares, the partial F, discarding *sex* from the complete model, will be:

$$F\left(sex \middle| age\right) = \frac{190.8/1}{239.3/7} = 5.58$$

And the partial F, again discarding *age* from the complete model, will be:

$$F\left(age \middle| sex\right) = \frac{43.2/1}{239.3/7} = 1.26$$

The respective null hypotheses are

$$H_0 : \beta_{sex|age} = 0$$

and

$$H_0 : \beta_{age|sex} = 0$$

The respective *P*-values are computed with the *F*-Fisher probability distribution with 1 and 7 degrees of freedom. In Stata, these *P*-values can be obtained using the *Ftail* command, as is illustrated in the following:

```
. dis Ftail(1,7,(282.536554 - 239.30065)/34.1858072)
0.29783641
. dis Ftail(1,7,(430.07574- 239.30065)/34.1858072)
0.05017009
```

An alternative procedure is to use the *test* command after the *reg* command for the complete model, as in the following:

```
quietly: reg bmi age sex
test sex
test age
```

Output

```
. test sex

( 1)   sex = 0

       F(   1,       7) =     5.58
               Prob > F =     0.0502

. test age

( 1)   age = 0

       F(   1,       7) =     1.26
               Prob > F =     0.2978
```

Thus, we conclude that there is marginal evidence against the null hypothesis, H_0: $\beta_{sex|age} = 0$ (*P*-value = .05), suggesting that the variable *sex* could be part of the model when the variable *age* is already one of the predictors.

5.13 Prediction

Should the user pursue using the model for predicting the expected value under the specific conditions of the predictors, the *adjust* command is available in Stata for this purpose. For example, assuming that the user is interested in estimating the expected bmi for females (sex = 1) aged 30 years; after the *reg* command, the specifications for the adjust command are as follows:

```
quietly: reg bmi age sex
adjust age=30 sex=1, ci
```

Output

```
----------------------------------------------------------------
    Dependent variable: bmi     Command: regress
Covariates set to value: age = 30, sex = 1
----------------------------------------------------------------

    ---------------------------------------------------------
    All |           xb             lb             ub
---------+-----------------------------------------------
        |     33.9999      [26.8742       41.1257]
    ---------------------------------------------------------
    Key:  xb      =   Linear Prediction
          [lb , ub]  =   [95% Confidence Interval]
```

The option *ci* in the adjust command is used to display the 95% confidence interval of the prediction. The results displayed in the above table indicate that for 30-year-old females, the estimated expected bmi is 34 (95% CI: 26.9, 41.1).

5.14 Polynomial Linear Regression Model

Another extension of the SLRM is the polynomial linear regression model, with at least one predictor at the power greater than 1. This model is recommended when it is suspected that a nonlinear trend would better explain the relationship between the outcome of interest and the predictors. The simplest polynomial model is the following expression:

$$Y_i = \beta_0 + \beta_1 X_i + \beta_2 X_i^2 + e_i$$

The model above is known as a second-order or quadratic polynomial model, because it contains an independent variable expressed as a term to the first power (X_i) and a term expressed to the second power (X_i^2). To use this model, it is recommended that all predictors be centralized to reduce the effect of the correlation among predictors. For example, to explain the variable *bmi* by *age* and *age²*, the following commands generate the estimates of the expected values for both the linear and polynomial models:

```
quietly: sum age
gen agec=age-r(mean)
gen agec2=agec^2
reg bmi agec
predict bmiesp1
reg bmi agec agec2
predict bmiesp2
```

Output

```
quietly: sum age
. gen agec=age-r(mean)
. gen agec2=agec^2
. reg bmi agec
```

Source	SS	df	MS		
Model	1.55497935	1	1.55497935		
Residual	430.075749	8	53.7594686		
Total	431.630728	9	47.9589698		

```
      Number of obs =      10
      F( 1,      8) =    0.03
      Prob > F      =  0.8692
      R-squared     =  0.0036
      Adj R-squared = -0.1209
      Root MSE      =  7.3321
```

bmi	Coef.	Std. Err.	t	P>|t|	[95% Conf. Interval]
agec	.0701375	.4123967	0.17	0.869	-.8808511 1.021126
_cons	28.45408	2.318609	12.27	0.000	23.10736 33.8008

```
. predict bmiesp1
(option xb assumed; fitted values)

. reg bmi agec agec2
```

Source	SS	df	MS		
Model	68.2219892	2	34.1109946		
Residual	363.408739	7	51.9155342		
Total	431.630728	9	47.9589698		

```
      Number of obs =      10
      F( 2,      7) =    0.66
      Prob > F      =  0.5476
      R-squared     =  0.1581
      Adj R-squared = -0.0825
      Root MSE      =  7.2052
```

bmi	Coef.	Std. Err.	t	P>|t|	[95% Conf. Interval]
agec	.7288876	.7086385	1.03	0.338	-.9467761 2.404551
agec2	-.0769584	.0679124	-1.13	0.294	-.2375457 .0836289
_cons	30.88673	3.130483	9.87	0.000	23.48432 38.28915

```
. predict bmiesp2
(option xb assumed; fitted values)
```

Once the expected value for each model is estimated with the command predict (bmiesp1 and bmiesp2), a plot with these estimates can be displayed with the following command (Figure 5.2):

```
twoway (scatter bmi age, sort) (line bmiesp1 age, sort) (line
bmiesp2 age, sort), ytitle(bmi)
```

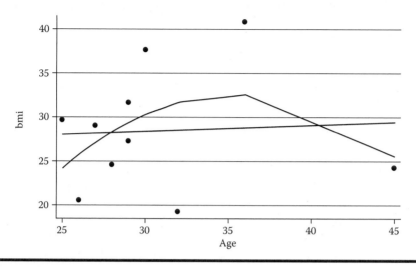

Figure 5.2   Linear and polynomial fits.

Output

In this example, the quadratic curve appears to be better than the linear trend in terms of its ability to explain the expected value of bmi by *age*.

5.15 Sample Size and Statistical Power

To determine the minimum sample size for performing an SLRM with enough statistical power (i.e., $1 - \beta = 0.8$) and a minimum significance level (i.e., $\alpha = 0.05$), the following expression is used (Kleinbaum et al., 2008):

$$n_s \geq \left[\frac{Z_{1-\frac{\alpha}{2}}+Z_{1-\beta}}{C(\rho)}\right]^2 + 3$$

in which $C(\rho)$ is the Fisher transformation, defined as follows:

$$C(\rho) = \frac{1}{2}\text{Ln}\left(\frac{1+\rho}{1-\rho}\right)$$

In the above, ρ can be estimated with the square root of the expected coefficient of determination (R^2) for the model under consideration.

In Stata we can estimate sample size using the option of correlation in the *Power and sample size analysis* window in the *Statistics* menu, providing significance level, power value, and the linear correlation coefficient value under the alternative

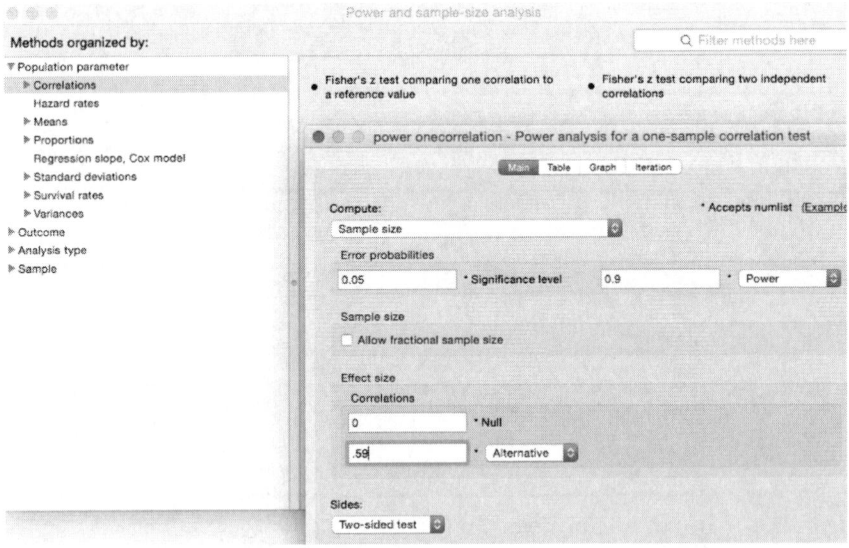

Figure 5.3 Power and sample-size analysis.

hypothesis. For example, assuming that we want to determine the minimum sample size needed to estimate the expected *bmi* value using an SLRM with sex as predictor and an approximate R^2 of 0.3454 ($\rho \sim \sqrt{.3454} = .59$), the dialog box should be filled out as described in Figure 5.3.

Output

```
Estimated sample size for a one-sample correlation test
Fisher's z test
Ho: r = r0   versus   Ha: r != r0

Study parameters:

        alpha =    0.0500
        power =    0.9000
        delta =    0.5900
           r0 =    0.0000
           ra =    0.5900
Estimated sample size:

          N =         26
```

Therefore, the minimum sample size for performing an SLRM between BMI and *sex*, assuming 90% statistical power and a 5% significance level, is 26 subjects. Should the user want to determine the minimum sample size for an MLRM (n_m), when X_1 is the main predictor, the following expression is recommended (Kleinbaum et al., 2008):

$$n_m = \frac{n_s}{1 - \rho^2_{X_1(X_2,\ldots,X_k)}}$$

where n_s is the minimum sample size for the SLRM using X_1 as predictor, $\rho^2_{X_1(X_2,\ldots,X_k)}$ is the chosen value of the population-squared multiple correlation between the main predictor X_1 and the control variables $X_2, X_3,\ldots,X_k$.

5.16 Considerations for the Assumptions of the Linear Regression Model

Having defined the linear regression model most suitable to your needs, it is necessary to verify its compliance with the assumptions for its creation. This assessment is conducted primarily through the absolute difference between the observed and expected values under the model:

$$\hat{e}_i = y_i - \hat{y}_i$$

where

$$\hat{y}_i = \hat{\beta}_0 + \hat{\beta}_1 X_1 + \cdots + \hat{\beta}_p X_p$$

At first it is assumed that the residuals are independent; however, the e_i obtained from the study data depend on the expected values of Y under the model, which in turn depend on the values of the predictors. Moreover, the model assumes that

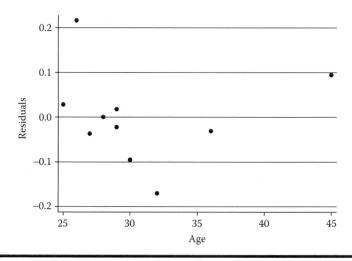

Figure 5.4 Residuals distribution.

the variances are constant, but the variance of the residual depends on the distance of the central values of the predictors. To verify the compliance of constant variance, it is recommended that the standardized residuals be graphically represented. In Stata, this type of graph can be obtained using the *rvpplot* command after the *reg* command. For example, to describe the residuals distribution related with the linear regression model between *heimt* and *age,* the Stata commands are:

```
reg heimt age
rvpplot age
```

The output of these commands can be seen in Figure 5.4. Because of the small sample size in this example, it is difficult to visualize a particular pattern around 0, although some symmetric distribution is observed. For more discussion on this topic, we recommend checking out the book by Draper and Smith (1998).

Chapter 6

Analysis of Variance

Aim: Upon completing the chapter, the learner should be able to perform an analysis of variance to compare the expected values of a continuous random variable between different groups.

6.1 Introduction

An analysis of variance (ANOVA) can be performed to compare two or more parameters (expected values and variances). The possible objectives of this analysis might be to:

1. Compare the expected value of a continuous random variable in "m" different groups to assess the following hypothesis:

$$H_0 : \mu_1 = \mu_2 = \cdots = \mu_m$$

2. Determine which expected values are different among comparison groups to evaluate any of the following potential null hypotheses:

$$H_0 : \mu_i = \mu_j; H_0 : \mu_i = \frac{\mu_i + \mu_k}{2}; H_0 : \frac{\mu_1 + \mu_2 + \mu_3}{3} = \frac{\mu_4 + \mu_5}{2} \cdots$$

3. Determine if the variability of a random continuous variable is the same between different groups to evaluate the following hypothesis:

$$H_0 : \sigma_\alpha^2 = 0$$

6.2 Data Structure

Assuming that we have three groups or three selected groups, the database to compare the expected value of random variable Y would have the following structure:

	Group 1	Group 2	Group 3	
	$Y_{1,1}$	$Y_{2,1}$	$Y_{3,1}$	
	$Y_{1,2}$	$Y_{2,2}$	$Y_{3,2}$	
	$\vdots$	$\vdots$	$\vdots$	
	$\vdots$	$\vdots$	$\vdots$	
	$Y_{1,n1}$	$Y_{2,n2}$	$Y_{3,n3}$	Total
Total	$\sum_{j=1}^{n1} Y_{1,j}$	$\sum_{j=1}^{n2} Y_{2,j}$	$\sum_{j=1}^{n3} Y_{3,j}$	$\sum_{i=1}^{k}\sum_{j=1}^{n_i} Y_{i,j}$
Mean	$\bar{Y}_1$	$\bar{Y}_2$	$\bar{Y}_3$	$\bar{Y}$
Variance	s_1^2	s_2^2	s_2^2	s^2
Number of subjects	n_1	n_2	n_3	n
Expected value	μ_1	μ_2	μ_3	μ

The possible research questions for this study are:

1. Assuming that the information available is from all possible groups, the research question can be stated as follows: Does the expected value vary by group ($\mu_1 = \mu_2 = \mu_3$)? (Fixed effects model)
2. Assuming that the information available is from a random sample of all possible groups, the research question can be stated as follows: Is there any variation among all the groups ($\sigma_\alpha^2 \neq 0$)? (Random effects model)

6.3 Example for Fixed Effects

To exemplify the research question for fixed effects (above), we are going to use the information from the previous database. As the *bmig* consists of three groups (normal, overweight, and obese), the research question would be the following: Are there differences in the expected age, according to the *bmig* categories?

The basic statistics from the database, using the *table* command, are in the following output:

```
. table bmig, c(n age mean age sd age)

------------------------------------------------
      bmig|    N(age)    mean(age)      sd(age)
----------+-------------------------------------
    Normal|         4        32.75     8.539125
Overweight|         3           27            2
     Obese|         3     31.66667     3.785939
------------------------------------------------
```

The results from the above table show that subjects having a normal bmi are in the older group, and those categorized as being overweight are younger. But the variability in these groups seems to be very different, based on the comparison of standard deviations. To assess whether these differences are statistically significant, either a linear model or an analysis of variance can be used (both of which are described in the following sections).

6.4 Linear Model with Fixed Effects

For a comparison of the expected values of a continuous random variable Y (e.g., age in years) for the groups of interest, we can establish the following model, using the bmig categories:

$$y_{ij} = \mu_1 + (\mu_2 - \mu_1) * \text{BMIG}_2 + (\mu_3 - \mu_1) * \text{BMIG}_3 + e_{ij}$$

and

$$y_{ij} = \mu_1 + \alpha_2 * \text{BMIG}_2 + \alpha_3 * \text{BMIG}_3 + e_{ij}$$

where:

y_{ij} indicates the value of the continuous random variable Y in the ith subject that belongs to the jth bmig category

μ_j indicates the expected value of Y in the jth *bmig* category, $E(y_{ij}) = \mu_j$

e_{ij} indicates the difference between the observed value of y_{ij} and the expected value of the random variable Y in the jth bmig category (μ_j) (it is assumed that the errors, e_{ij}, are independent and follow an $N(0, \sigma^2)$ distribution)

α_j indicates the effect of the jth *bmig* category with respect to the first bmig category (normal), subject to the restriction $\alpha_1 = 0$

BMIG_j is a dummy variable whose value is 1 if the subject belongs to the jth bmig category; its value is 0 if the subject belongs to another bmig group

When the groups being compared correspond to all of the possible groups or when they represent a select group of interest, the α_is are constants and are defined as fixed effects. If the effects are fixed, then it is initially assumed that variances within groups are equal, $\text{Var}(Y_{ij}) = \sigma^2$.

6.5 Analysis of Variance with Fixed Effects

For analyzing the expected values of a continuous random variable between different groups using the statistical method of analysis of variance, we start by decomposing the numerator of the variance of Y, as can be accomplished using the following:

$$\sum_{i=1}^{k}\sum_{j=1}^{n_i}(Y_{ij}-\bar{Y})^2 = \sum_{i=1}^{k}n_i(\bar{Y}_i-\bar{Y})^2 + \sum_{i=1}^{k}\sum_{j=1}^{n_i}(Y_{ij}-\bar{Y}_i)^2$$

where:

$\sum_{i=1}^{k}n_i(\bar{Y}_i-\bar{Y})^2$ indicates the variation between groups (*between sum of squares*)
$\sum_{i=1}^{k}\sum_{j=1}^{n_i}(Y_{ij}-\bar{Y})^2$ indicates the overall variation within each group (*within sum of squares*)

The null hypothesis in ANOVA with fixed effects determines that the expected values of the random variable of interest, Y, in all groups are the same, $H_0 : \mu_1 = \cdots = \mu_k$; thus, $\alpha_i = 0$ for all groups. To assess the null hypothesis, the estimated expected values of SS between and SS within are compared, considering their respective degrees of freedom, as follows:

Source of Variation	SS	Df	MS	E[MS]
Between	$\sum_{i=1}^{k}n_i(\bar{Y}_i-\bar{Y})^2$	$k-1$	$\sum_{i=1}^{k}n_i(\bar{Y}_i-\bar{Y})^2/(k-1)$	$\sigma^2+\phi$
Within	$\sum_{i=1}^{k}\sum_{j=1}^{n_i}(Y_{ij}-\bar{Y}_i)^2$	$n-k$	$\sum_{i=1}^{k}\sum_{j=1}^{n_i}(Y_{ij}-\bar{Y}_i)^2/(n-k)$	σ^2
Total	$\sum_{i=1}^{k}\sum_{j=1}^{n_i}(Y_{ij}-\bar{Y})^2$	$n-1$		

Note: $\phi = \dfrac{1}{k-1}\sum_{i=1}^{k}n_i\alpha_i^2$

Under the null hypotheses, the ratio $\left(\sigma^2 + \frac{1}{k-1}\sum n_i\alpha_i^2 \big/ \sigma^2\right) = 1$. To determine how far this ratio should be away from 1, once a dataset is collected and the parameters of the linear model $\left(\sigma^2, \alpha_i\right)$ are estimated, a *P*-value is computed using the *F*-Fisher probability distribution with 1 and *n* – 2 degrees of freedom.

6.6 Programming for ANOVA

To program a linear model to determine which fixed effect is different from zero, we can use the *regress* (or *reg*) command with a categorical predictor. For example, to compare age between the categories of the bmig, using the first category as the reference group, go to the *Statistics* dropdown menu and click on "Linear regression"; next, write *age* in the Dependent variable box and *bmig* (as a categorical variable) in the Independent variables box, remembering to precede "bmig" with the symbol "*i.*", as is illustrated in Figure 6.1.

Once the previous table is submitted, the following output will be displayed:

```
. reg  age i.bmig

      Source |       SS          df       MS          Number of obs =        10
-------------+----------------------------------      F(2, 7)       =      0.83
       Model | 60.6833333        2   30.3416667       Prob > F      =    0.4742
    Residual | 255.416667        7   36.4880952       R-squared     =    0.1920
-------------+----------------------------------      Adj R-squared =   -0.0389
       Total |      316.1        9   35.1222222       Root MSE      =    6.0405
```

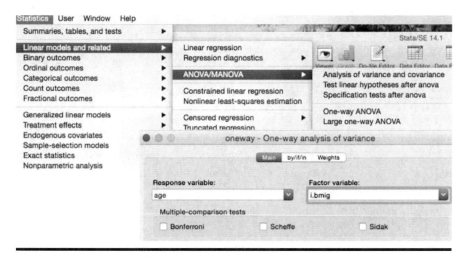

Figure 6.1   Linear regression model with categorical predictor.

```
-----------------------------------------------------------------------------
       age |     Coef.   Std. Err.      t    P>|t|    [95% Conf. Interval]
-----------+-----------------------------------------------------------------
      bmig |
Overweight |     -5.75   4.613537   -1.25    0.253    -16.65928    5.159281
     Obese | -1.083333   4.613537   -0.23    0.821    -11.99261    9.825948
           |
     _cons |     32.75   3.020269   10.84    0.000      25.6082    39.8918
-----------------------------------------------------------------------------
```

The results show that there is no evidence of significant differences in the mean age across bmig categories using normal subjects as the reference group (P-value > .1). If the user wants to change the reference group (e.g., use the second category of bmig), the following command syntax should be used:

`reg age b2.bmig`

Output

```
. reg  age b2.bmig

    Source |       SS         df       MS            Number of obs   =        10
-----------+------------------------------            F(2, 7)         =      0.83
     Model |  60.6833333      2    30.3416667         Prob > F        =    0.4742
  Residual |  255.416667      7    36.4880952         R-squared       =    0.1920
-----------+------------------------------            Adj R-squared   =   -0.0389
     Total |       316.1      9    35.1222222         Root MSE        =    6.0405


-----------------------------------------------------------------------------
       age |     Coef.   Std. Err.      t    P>|t|    [95% Conf. Interval]
-----------+-----------------------------------------------------------------
      bmig |
    Normal |      5.75   4.613537    1.25    0.253    -5.159281    16.65928
     Obese |  4.666667   4.932078    0.95    0.376    -6.995845    16.32918
           |
     _cons |        27   3.487506    7.74    0.000     18.75336    35.24664
-----------------------------------------------------------------------------
```

The commands *oneway* and *anova* can be used in the assessment of the null hypothesis, $H_0 : \mu_1 = \cdots = \mu_k$ (using fixed-effect ANOVA). The *oneway* command includes Bartlett's test for equal variances, a condition needed in the F-test for comparing expected values. The *anova* command expands the sum of squares if more than one source of variation is used. For example, to compare age between the bmig categories, the following command is used:

`oneway age bmig`

Output

```
. oneway age bmig
```

<table>
<tr><th colspan="7">Analysis of Variance</th></tr>
<tr><th>Source</th><th>SS</th><th>df</th><th>MS</th><th>F</th><th colspan="2">Prob > F</th></tr>
<tr><td>Between groups</td><td>60.6833333</td><td>2</td><td>30.3416667</td><td>0.83</td><td colspan="2">0.4742</td></tr>
<tr><td>Within groups</td><td>255.416667</td><td>7</td><td>36.4880952</td><td></td><td></td><td></td></tr>
<tr><td>Total</td><td>316.1</td><td>9</td><td>35.1222222</td><td></td><td></td><td></td></tr>
</table>

```
Bartlett's test for equal variances: chi2(2) = 3.5156 Prob>chi2 = 0.172
```

The output of the *oneway* command provides evidence in favor of the null hypothesis, $H_0 : \mu_{normal} = \mu_{overweight} = \mu_{obese}$, and evidence in favor of equal variances, via the Bartlett's test (*P*-value > 0.1).

If the user includes the variable *sex* as a second source of variation and the interaction of *age* and *sex* to explore how the mean of *age* changes by bmig category and *sex*, the command line (making use of the *anova* command) is as follows:

```
anova age bmig sex bmig#sex
```

Output

```
                Number of obs =          10    R-squared     =   0.8439
                Root MSE      =     3.14113    Adj R-squared =   0.7191
```

Source	Partial SS	df	MS	F	Prob>F
Model	266.76667	4	66.691667	6.76	0.0299
bmig	157.11373	2	78.556863	7.96	0.0279
sex	131.92157	1	131.92157	13.37	0.0146
bmig#sex	62.745098	1	62.745098	6.36	0.0531
Residual	49.333333	5	9.8666667		
Total	316.1	9	35.122222		

The output suggests that the mean of *age* changes according to the *bmig* and *sex* categories due to the fact that the interaction term bmig#sex is marginally significant (*P*-value = .053); however, caution should be taken with this interpretation because the sample size is very small.

6.7 Planned Comparisons (before Observing the Data)

Having determined that there is evidence of a difference between the expected values, the next step is to determine if the difference of interest is significant. This difference of interest can be defined with two expected values (pairs of means) or with a combination of expected values (linear contrasts).

6.7.1 Comparison of Two Expected Values

Continuing with the same example as before, suppose the user's main purpose is to compare the expected age of subjects having a normal bmi with the expected age of subjects who are categorized as being overweight. To do this, the null hypothesis is formulated in the following way:

$$H_0 : \mu_1 = \mu_2 \quad \text{or} \quad H_0 : \mu_1 - \mu_2 = 0$$

which is equivalent to

$$H_0 : \alpha_2 = 0$$

The test statistic will be

$$F = t^2 = \left(\frac{\left| \bar{Y}_i - \bar{Y}_j \right|}{\sqrt{s^2 \left[\left(1/n_i \right) + \left(1/n_j \right) \right]}} \right)^2 \sim F_{1,n-k|H_0}$$

where s^2 is MSE (within MS).

To evaluate the null hypothesis in Stata, using this statistic, we can use the *test* command after the *anova* command, as can be seen in the following:

```
anova age bmig

test 1.bmig=2.bmig
```

Output

```
. anova age bmig

              Number of obs =        10    R-squared     =   0.1920
              Root MSE      = 6.04054    Adj R-squared = -0.0389

     Source |  Partial SS   df          MS          F         Prob>F
  ----------+--------------------------------------------------------
      Model |  60.683333    2    30.341667       0.83         0.4742

       bmig |  60.683333    2    30.341667       0.83         0.4742

   Residual |  255.41667    7    36.488095
  ----------+--------------------------------------------------------
      Total |     316.1     9    35.122222
```

```
.   test 1.bmig=2.bmig

 ( 1)  1b.bmig  -  2.bmig  =  0

      F(   1,        7) =      1.55
             Prob > F =      0.2527
```

The results suggest that there is no difference in the expected age between normal bmi subjects and those whose bmi indicates that they are overweight (*P*-value > .1).

6.7.2 Linear Contrast

A linear contrast is a combination of expected values, as is illustrated in the following:

$$L = \sum_{i=1}^{k} c_i \mu_i$$

where:

$$\sum_{i=1}^{k} c_i = 0$$

The definition for a linear contrast depends on the null hypothesis under evaluation. For example,

1. When $H_0 : \mu_1 - \mu_2 = 0$ then,

$$L = (1)\mu_1 + (-1)\mu_2$$

   where $c_1 = 1$ and $c_2 = -1$

2. When $H_0 : \mu_1 = (\mu_2 + \mu_3/2) \Rightarrow H_0 : (1)\mu_1 + (-0.5)\mu_2 + (-0.5)\mu_3 = 0$ then,

$$L = (1)\mu_1 + (-0.5)\mu_2 + (-0.5)\mu_3$$

   where $c_1 = 1$, $c_2 = -0.5$, $c_3 = -0.5$

Once the linear contrast is defined, the test statistic is

$$t = \frac{\hat{L}}{\sqrt{s^2 \sum_{i=1}^{k} \left(c_i^2 / n_i \right)}} \sim t_{\left(n-k, 1-\frac{\alpha}{2} \right)}$$

where s^2 = MSE (within MS) and $\hat{L}$ is determined by the sample means.

To evaluate linear contrasts in Stata, we can use the *test* command after the *anova* command. For example, assuming the user wants to compare the expected age between the subjects categorized as having a normal bmi against the average of the expected age in subjects categorized as being overweight or obese, the null hypothesis is formulated as H_0: $\mu_1 = (\mu_2 + \mu_3)/2$. To assess this hypothesis with the *test* command, the specified command line, after running the *anova* command, is as follows:

```
test 1.bmig=(2.bmig+3.bmig)/2
```

Output

```
. test 1.bmig=(2.bmig+3.bmig)/2
 ( 1)   1b.bmig - .5*2.bmig - .5*3.bmig = 0
        F(  1,    7) =    0.77
             Prob > F =    0.4099
```

The results suggest that the expected age does not change between the groups under comparison (*P*-value > .1).

6.8 Multiple Comparisons: Unplanned Comparisons

Having determined that there is evidence of a difference between the expected values, the next step is to determine which of the differences is or are significant. There are several methods, called post hoc tests, which have been developed to answer this type of question; two of the most commonly used methods are *Bonferroni's method* and *Scheffé's method*.

Bonferroni's method compares pairs of groups by adjusting the significance level of each pair of averages compared to the total possible number of paired comparisons. For example, if the level of significance is 5% and there are three possible pairwise comparisons, then the level of significance for evaluating one particular pair of means is divided by 3; that is, the level of significance of one pair would be $0.05/3 = 0.0167$. Another alternative is to multiply the *P*-value of each comparison by 3. This method ensures that the overall significance level defined in ANOVA is maintained when it is conducted simultaneously on all possible pairwise comparisons. This method can be programmed through the *oneway* command. For example, assuming the user wants to compare the expected age in the following three bmig categories (normal, overweight, and obese), the command syntax with *oneway* command will be the following:

```
oneway age bmig, bon tab
```

Output

bmig	Summary of age		
	Mean	Std. Dev.	Freq.
Normal	32.75	8.5391256	4
Overweigh	27	2	3
Obese	31.666667	3.7859389	3
Total	30.7	5.9264004	10

```
                        Analysis of Variance
      Source                SS           df        MS          F      Prob > F
    ------------------------------------------------------------------------
    Between groups      60.6833333        2    30.3416667   0.83      0.4742
    Within groups      255.416667         7    36.4880952

    ------------------------------------------------------------------------
       Total                         316.1     9    35.1222222
```

Bartlett's test for equal variances: chi2(2) = 3.5156 Prob>chi2 = 0.172

```
                                Comparison of age by bmig
                                       (Bonferroni)
    Row Mean-|
    Col Mean |       Normal    Overweig
    ---------+-----------------------------
    Overweig |       -5.75
             |        0.758
             |
       Obese |     -1.08333     4.66667
             |      1.000        1.000
```

Note: The option Bon displays the Bonferroni multiple-comparison test. The option tab produces a summary of age at each category of bmig.

At the bottom of the output table, all the pairwise comparisons between the samples means can be seen; for example, the difference between the mean age of the obese group and that of the overweight group is 4.67, which can be confirmed with the first table requested in this output, in which $\bar{Y}_{normal} = 32.8$, $\bar{Y}_{overweight} = 27.0$, and $\bar{Y}_{obese} = 31.7$. Below the pairwise differences is the *P*-value for the *F*-statistics of one pair, which was computed by multiplying by the total number of possible mean pairs to be compared. The results show that there are no evidences of significant differences (*P*-values > .1) in any of the pairwise comparisons.

Scheffé's method performs multiple comparisons through linear contrasts, but the significance level of each comparison is not adjusted. In Scheffé's method, the test statistic is calculated using the following formula:

$$t^2 / (k-1) = \left(\frac{\hat{L}}{\sqrt{s^2 \sum_{i=1}^{k} \left(c_i^2 / n_i \right)}} \right)^2 / (k-1)$$

The null hypothesis is rejected with a certain significance level, α, when

$$t > \sqrt{(k-1) F_{k-1, n-k, 1-\alpha}} \quad \text{or} \quad t < -\sqrt{(k-1) F_{k-1, n-k, 1-\alpha}}$$

The *P*-value is calculated with the *F*-Fisher probability distribution with $k - 1$ and $n - k$ degrees of freedom. The Stata command line for performing multiple comparisons by Scheffé's method is as follows:

```
oneway age bmig, sch
```

Output

```
**The ANOVA table is omitted
Comparison of age by bmig
                                    (Scheffe)
Row Mean-|
Col Mean |      Normal   Overweig
---------+-----------------------------
Overweig |      -5.75
         |      0.496
         |
   Obese |    -1.08333    4.66667
         |      0.973      0.656
```

The results displayed in the above output table show that the *P*-values that result when using Scheffé's method are different from those that result when Bonferroni's method is used; however, the statistical evidence confirms that there are no significant differences (*P*-values > .1) in any of the pairwise comparisons.

6.9 Random Effects

When the statistical information is collected only from a random sample of groups of subjects, which are part of all possible study groups (Figure 6.2), we can define a linear model with random effects.

The linear model with random effects is represented as follows:

```
Yij|μi = μi + eij,
```

where:
$$Y_{ij}|\mu_i \sim \text{i.i.d } N\left(\mu_i, \sigma^2\right)$$
$$\mu_i \sim \text{i.i.d } N\left(\mu_i, \sigma_\mu^2\right)$$
i.i.d = independently and identically distributed

The main outcome, *Y*, is a continuous random variable distributed as a normal distribution with the following parameters: μ_i, σ^2. These parameters could be also random variables; however, in the random effect model considered, only μ_i is assumed to be a random variable with normal distribution and parameters: μ, σ_μ^2.

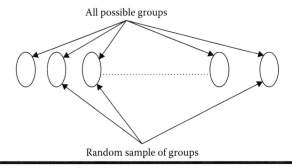

Figure 6.2 Random effects scheme.

Following is an alternative expression of the linear model with random effects:

$$E\left(Y_{ij}|\alpha_i\right) = \mu + \alpha_i$$

$$Y_{ij}|\alpha_i \sim \text{i.i.d}\, N\left(\mu_i, \sigma^2\right)$$

$$\alpha_i \sim \text{i.i.d}\, N\left(0, \sigma_\alpha^2\right)$$

The procedure to estimate the parameters of this model is similar to the process used in Bayesian data analysis; however, in ANOVA with random effects, we are only assuming randomness in μ_i. The null hypothesis of the ANOVA with random effects is formulated as follows:

$$H_0 : \sigma_\alpha^2 = 0$$

Having $\sigma_\alpha^2 = 0$ implies that the expected values of Y for all groups, including the groups in the study sample and the groups of subjects who were not included in the study sample, are equal $\left(\mu_1 = \mu_2 = \cdots = \mu_m\right)$.

Under the assumption of random effects, the expected values for the sum of squares in the ANOVA can be seen below in the following:

Source of Variation	SS	Df	MS	E[MS]
Between	$\sum_{i=1}^{k} n_i\left(\bar{Y}_i - \bar{Y}\right)^2$	$k - 1$	$\sum_{i=1}^{k} n_i\left(\bar{Y}_i - \bar{Y}\right)^2 / (k-1)$	$\sigma^2 + n_0 \sigma_\alpha^2$
Within	$\sum_{i=1}^{k}\sum_{j=1}^{n_i}\left(Y_{ij} - \bar{Y}_i\right)^2$	$n - k$	$\sum_{i=1}^{k}\sum_{j=1}^{n_i}\left(Y_{ij} - \bar{Y}_i\right)^2 / (n-k)$	σ^2
Total	$\sum_{i=1}^{k}\sum_{j=1}^{n_i}\left(Y_{ij} - \bar{Y}\right)^2$	$n - 1$		

where:

$$n_0 = \frac{\sum_{i=1}^{k} n_i - \left[\left(\sum_{i=1}^{k} n_i^2 \middle/ \sum_{i=1}^{k} n_i \right) \right]}{k-1}$$

According to the null hypothesis $\left(H_0 : \sigma_\alpha^2 = 0 \right)$,

$$\frac{E \left(MS_{Between} \right)}{E \left(MS_{Within} \right)} = 1$$

To evaluate the null hypothesis with the data collected in the sample, the F-statistic is obtained using the following equation:

$$F = \frac{\sum_{i=1}^{k} n_i \left(\bar{Y}_i - \bar{Y} \right)^2 / (k-1)}{\sum_{i=1}^{k} \sum_{j=1}^{n_i} \left(Y_{ij} - \bar{Y}_i \right)^2 / (n-k)} \sim F_{(k-1, n-k, 1-\alpha)}$$

The estimates of σ_α^2 and σ^2 are calculated by the following expressions:

$$\widehat{\sigma_\alpha^2} = \max \left(\frac{MS_{Between} - MS_{Within}}{n_0}, 0 \right)$$

$$\hat{\sigma}^2 = \sum_{i=1}^{k} \sum_{j=1}^{n_i} \frac{\left(Y_{ij} - \bar{Y}_i \right)^2}{(n-k)}$$

6.10 Other Measures Related to the Random Effects Model

6.10.1 Covariance

In the previous example, there is a possible relationship between the subjects of the same group. To assess this, the covariance statistic is defined using the following equation:

$$\text{Cov}(Y_{im}, Y_{in}) = \text{Cov}\{E(Y_{im}|\alpha_i, E(Y_{in}|\alpha_i)\} + E\{\text{Cov}(Y_{im}, Y_{in}|\alpha_i)\}$$
$$= \text{Cov}(\mu + \alpha_i, \mu + \alpha_i) + 0 = \text{Cov}(\alpha_i, \alpha_i) = \sigma_\alpha^2$$

6.10.2 Variance and Its Components

Another expression for the variance of Y_{ij} with its components is as follows:

$$\text{Var}(Y_{ij}) = \text{Var}\{E(Y_{ij}|\alpha_i)\} + E\{\text{Var}(Y_{ij}|\alpha_i)\}$$
$$= \text{Var}(\mu + \alpha_i) + E(\sigma^2) = \sigma_\alpha^2 + \sigma^2$$

where σ_α^2 and σ^2 are defined as components of the variance.

6.10.3 Intraclass Correlation Coefficient

A useful measure of association within groups is the intraclass correlation coefficient defined as follows:

$$\text{Corr}(Y_{ij}, Y_{il}) = \frac{\text{Cov}(Y_{ij}, Y_{il})}{\sqrt{\text{Var}(Y_{ij})\text{Var}(Y_{il})}} = \frac{\sigma_\alpha^2}{\sqrt{(\sigma_\alpha^2 + \sigma^2)(\sigma_\alpha^2 + \sigma^2)}} = \frac{\sigma_\alpha^2}{\sigma_\alpha^2 + \sigma^2} = \rho_I$$

This index can be interpreted as a measure of reproducibility or consistency (reliability coefficient) between the measurements of a group. Rosner (2010) suggests using the following interpretations:

$\rho_I < 0.4$	Poor reproducibility
$0.4 \le \rho_I < 0.75$	Moderate reproducibility
$\rho_I \ge 0.75$	Excellent reproducibility

6.11 Example of a Random Effects Model

Let us assume that the user is interested in assessing the systolic blood pressure readings (mm Hg) from a portable machine. In addition, we must take into consideration the fact that the experimental design was defined to measure these readings from a subject twice a day, for 10 consecutive days, as a random sample of days in 1 month. Finally, let us assume that the data in Stata conform to the following format:

```
     +-------------------+
     | day   sb1    sb2  |
     |-------------------|
 1.  |  1     98     99  |
 2.  |  2    102     93  |
 3.  |  3    100     98  |
 4.  |  4     99    100  |
 5.  |  5     96    100  |
 6.  |  6     95    100  |
 7.  |  7     90     98  |
 8.  |  8    102     93  |
 9.  |  9     91     92  |
10.  | 10     90     94  |
     +-------------------+
     sb1 indicates the first measure of systolic blood pressure.
     sb2 indicates the second measure of systolic blood pressure.
```

To perform an ANOVA, the user has to modify the previous database structure. The actual format is called *wide* format, where every row in the dataset contains all the information of one subject. To run an ANOVA the database structure must be in the *long* format, where every row contains the information of each subject's visit. The **reshape** command can be used to change the database structure from *wide* to *long* format, as follows:

```
reshape long sb, i(day)
```

Output

```
. reshape long sb, i(day)
(note: j = 1 2)

Data                                   wide   ->   long
-------------------------------------------------------------
Number of obs.                           10   ->     20
Number of variables                       3   ->      3
j variable (2 values)                          ->     _j
xij variables:
                                    sb1 sb2   ->     sb
-------------------------------------------------------------
```

After the *reshape* command, use the *list* command to see the current data structure, as is demonstrated in the following table:

```
list
      +----------------+
   i  |  day   _j   sb |
      |----------------|
   1. |   1    1    98 |
   2. |   1    2    99 |
   3. |   2    1   102 |
   4. |   2    2    93 |
   5. |   3    1   100 |
   6. |   3    2    98 |
   7. |   4    1    99 |
   8. |   4    2   100 |
   9. |   5    1    96 |
  10. |   5    2   100 |
  11. |   6    1    95 |
  12. |   6    2   100 |
  13. |   7    1    90 |
  14. |   7    2    98 |
  15. |   8    1   102 |
  16. |   8    2    93 |
  17. |   9    1    91 |
  18. |   9    2    92 |
  19. |  10    1    90 |
  20. |  10    2    94 |
      +----------------+
```

To run the linear model with random effects, use the *loneway* command, as follows:

```
loneway sb day
```

Output

```
        One-way Analysis of Variance for sb:

                                         Number of obs =        20
                                         R-squared =        0.5118

   Source              SS        df      MS            F      Prob > F
-----------------------------------------------------------------------
Between day           152        9      16.888889     1.16    0.4050
Within day            145       10      14.5
-----------------------------------------------------------------------
Total                 297       19      15.631579

        Intraclass      Asy.
        correlation     S.E.     [95% Conf. Interval]
        --------------------------------------------------
            0.07611     0.32301      0.00000      0.70920

        Estimated SD of day effect            1.092906
        Estimated SD within day               3.807887
        Est. reliability of a day mean        0.14145
             (evaluated at n=2.00)
```

The results indicate that there is evidence in favor of the null hypothesis $\left(H_0 : \sigma_\alpha^2 = 0\right)$. Therefore, the expected values of the systolic blood pressure readings from the portable machine are equal for the subject under study for 1 month (P-value > .1). The estimated intraclass correlation coefficient is as follows:

$$\widehat{\rho}_I = \frac{1.19}{1.19 + 14.5} = 0.076$$

where $\widehat{\sigma}_\alpha^2 = (16.9 - 14.5/2) = 1.19$. Therefore, based on the intraclass correlation coefficient estimation, there is a poor reproducibility index between the two measurements taken in a single day.

6.12 Sample Size and Statistical Power

To determine the minimum sample size for comparing means with enough statistical power (i.e., at least $1 - \beta = 0.8$) and a minimum significance level (i.e., $\alpha = 0.05$), Stata provides the option for comparing the means of independent samples using ANOVA with the *Power and sample size analysis* window in the *Statistics* menu. For example, assuming we want to determine the minimum sample size to compare their mean age across the three bmig categories, the following information must be provided in the option *One-way analysis of variance*: significance level, statistical power, the group of means under the alternative hypothesis, and the error (within-group) variance (Figure 6.3).

Once the previous table is submitted, the following output will be displayed:

```
. power oneway 32.8   27 31.7, varerror(36.5)

Performing iteration ...

Estimated sample size for one-way ANOVA
F test for group effect
Ho: delta = 0   versus   Ha: delta != 0

Study parameters:

        alpha =    0.0500
        power =    0.8000
        delta =    0.4163
          N_g =         3
           m1 =   32.8000
           m2 =   27.0000
           m3 =   31.7000
        Var_m =    6.3267
        Var_e =   36.5000
```

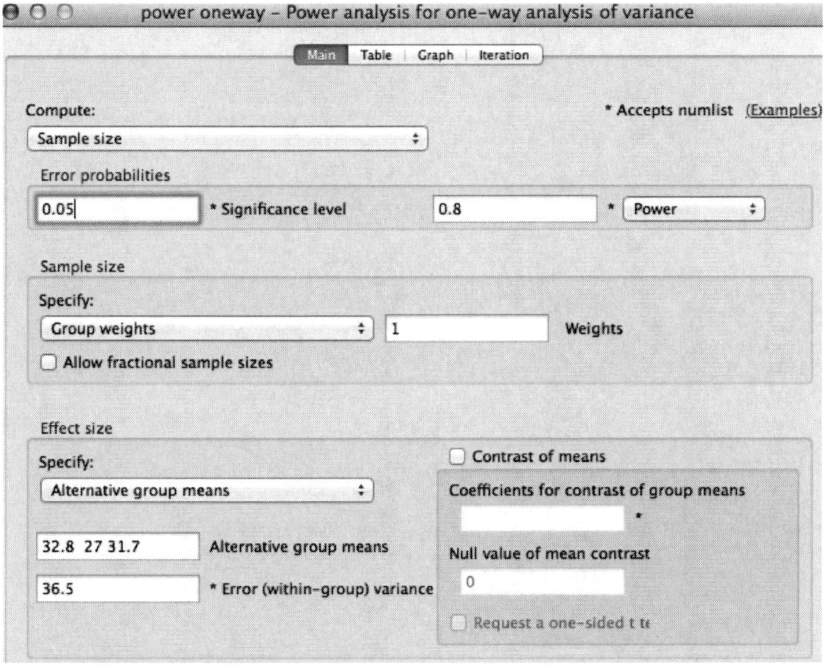

Figure 6.3 Sample size for one-way ANOVA.

```
Estimated sample sizes:

            N =           60
N per group =           20
```

Both delta (effect design, $\sqrt{\text{Var\_m}}/\sqrt{\text{Var\_e}}$) and Var_m (variance between groups, based on the means of each group and the grand mean, $\sum_{i=1}^{3}\left[\left(\overline{Y}_i - \overline{Y}\right)^2/3\right]$) are computed automatically by Stata.

Therefore, the minimum sample size to compare the means across the three bmig categories is 20 subjects per group, assuming the following conditions: an 80% statistical power, a 5% significance level, and an error (within-group) variance of 36.5.

Chapter 7

Categorical Data Analysis

Aim: Upon completing the chapter, the learner should be able to perform a stratified analysis in an epidemiological study, using cohort and case-control study designs.

7.1 Introduction

So far, we have discussed the Stata commands for estimating the conditional expectations of continuous variables. There are, however, numerous occasions in the public health field in which we are interested in exploring the association between a categorical outcome (e.g., disease status) and one or more predictor variables (e.g., exposure status, confounding variables, and effect modifiers variables) collected in epidemiologic studies. *Epidemiology* is "the study of the occurrence and distribution of health-related events in specified populations and the application of this knowledge to control relevant health problems" (Porta, 2008; Rothman, 2002). Epidemiological studies are commonly categorized as descriptive or analytical studies. These studies are defined immediately below:

- *Descriptive epidemiology* focuses on describing the occurrence (incidence, prevalence, and mortality) and distribution of disease (or other health event) patterns by characteristics relating to person (who is affected by the health event?), time (when does the health event occur?), and place (where does the health event occur?). Descriptive studies often use routine data (i.e., vital statistics, surveillance systems, registries, or population surveys) collected in a population to characterize the patterns of disease occurrence. The data generated from descriptive studies can be used for healthcare planning and hypothesis generation. Types of descriptive studies include case series, cross-sectional, and ecological studies.

■ *Analytical epidemiology* is concerned with assessing the associations between exposures and diseases (or other health outcomes), which associations may provide further insights into the causes of a disease and lead to prevention strategies. Types of analytical studies include case-control studies, cohort studies, and clinical trials.

In the next sections, we will show the application of the Mantel–Haenszel method for the analysis of data derived from cohort and case-control studies (Jewell, 2004; Rothman, 2002). This method is based on the stratification of potential confounding variables to estimate a weighted average of the magnitude of the exposure–disease association. Confounding factors are variables that are related to both the exposure and the outcome but do not lie in the causal pathway between them (Rothman, 2002; Woodward, 2004). As we shall see in the next chapters, regression models are efficient techniques that can be employed to assess the exposure–disease association while controlling for the *confounding variables*.

7.2 Cohort Study

Cohort studies are designed with at least two groups of subjects usually called *exposed* and *nonexposed* (in terms of a particular factor, in either case) groups. Once these groups are identified, they are followed up for a specific period of time to determine whether any of their members develop the disease of interest, while controlling for potential confounding variables. The magnitude of the association between *exposure* and *disease* is determined by the *relative risk*, which is defined in the following way:

$$RR = \frac{I_{exposure}}{I_{nonexposure}}$$

where I_j indicates the incidence of the disease in the *j*th group. When stratified analysis is performed, the RR is assessed under different strata (to be combined into one single RR) or reported in each stratum. In the *Mantel–Haenszel* method, the combined RR is computed using the weighted mean of the RRs, as follows:

$$RR_{M-H} = \sum \frac{w_k RR_k}{w_k}$$

where w_k is the weighted factor in the *k*th stratum, which is itself determined with the product of the total number of cases who are unexposed and the proportion of exposure in this stratum.

For example, let us say that we want to evaluate the association between alcohol intake (exposure) and a diagnosis of myocardial infarction (MI) over a period of 5 years, controlling for the effect of cigarette smoking (potential confounding variable). To analyze this type of study in Stata, we can use the following data:

	Smoker (0)		
Alcohol	MI + (1)	MI – (0)	Total
Present (1)	8	16	24
Absence (0)	22	44	66
Total	30	60	90
	Nonsmoker (1)		
Alcohol	MI + (1)	MI – (0)	Total
Present (1)	63	36	99
Absence (0)	7	4	11
Total	70	40	110

Between the parentheses are the codes for each category (1 indicates presence and 0 indicates absence).

To program these data, the database can be entered in Stata as follows:

```
    +----------------------------------+
    | smoker   alcohol   mi   subjects |
    |----------------------------------|
 1. |    0        1      1        8     |
 2. |    0        1      0       16     |
 3. |    0        0      1       22     |
 4. |    0        0      0       44     |
 5. |    1        1      1       63     |
 6. |    1        1      0       36     |
 7. |    1        0      1        7     |
 8. |    1        0      0        4     |
    +----------------------------------+
```

The command to perform a stratified analysis using the Mantel–Haenszel method is *cs*, as is illustrated in the following:

```
cs mi alcohol [fw=subjects], by (smoker)
```

Output

```
         smoker |    RR      [95% Conf. Interval]   M-H Weight
----------------+------------------------------------------------
              0 |     1     0.5164877   1.936154    5.866667
              1 |     1     0.6244517   1.601405    6.3
----------------+------------------------------------------------
          Crude | 1.53266   1.10769     2.120674
   M-H combined |     1     0.6695272   1.493591
----------------+------------------------------------------------
Test of homogeneity (M-H)   chi2(1) = 0.000   Pr>chi2 = 1.0000
```

Note: When the database collapses and contains a variable that tells the frequency of each observation, the *fw* option is used. This option specifies the variable that contains the number of times the observation was actually observed.

The output reports the point estimation of the relative risk (RR) for each stratum, as well as the crude RR and the weighted RR (RR$_{M-H}$) with their respective 95% confidence intervals. In addition, the weighted factor in each stratum is reported (M–H weight), as is the significance test (test of homogeneity [$H_0 : RR_1 = RR_2 = \cdots = RR_k$]), to assess whether the RRs in all strata are equal.

The results indicate that there is a nonsignificant difference in the RRs, per stratum (*P*-value > .10); therefore, it is recommended that the RR$_{M-H}$ be used. When we compare the point estimates of the crude $\widehat{RR} = 1.53$ and the $\widehat{RR}_{M-H} = 1$, we are able to conclude that the data show a strong confounding effect, as the crude RR is overestimating the magnitude of the association between MI and alcohol intake. Finally, the estimated magnitude of the association of interest, controlling for smoking, is 1 (95% CI: 0.67, 1.49); this, however, is not statistically significant (*P*-value > .05).

7.3 Case-Control Study

Case-control studies are designed initially with at least two groups of subjects, called *cases* (diseased) and *controls* (nondiseased). Once these groups are identified as having been exposed (or not) to a specific factor, they are then classified as being either exposed or nonexposed groups. The magnitude of the association between exposure and disease is determined by the *odds ratio* (OR), which is calculated with the following expression:

$$OR = \frac{Odds_{exposure}}{Odds_{nonexposure}}$$

where Odds$_j$ indicates the expected number of cases per control in the *j*th group (exposed or nonexposed) and can be defined as follows:

$$Odds = \frac{p}{1-p}$$

where *p* is the probability of having a diagnosis of the disease of interest under the study design.

In the Mantel–Haenszel method, the combined OR is computed using the weighted mean of the ORs, as follows:

$$OR_{M-H} = \sum \frac{w_k OR_k}{w_k}$$

where w_k is the weighted factor in the kth stratum, which is determined with the product of the number of cases who are unexposed and the number of controls who are exposed divided by the number of subjects in this stratum.

For example, let us assume that the user wants to evaluate the association between HPV (human papilloma virus) infection status and oropharyngeal cancer (OC), stratified by smoking (smokers vs. nonsmokers), using a case-control design with the following data:

Smoker (0)			
HPV	OC + (1)	OC – (0)	*Total*
Present (1)	75	20	95
Absent (0)	5	80	85
Total	80	100	180
Nonsmoker (1)			
HPV	OC + (1)	OC – (0)	*Total*
Present (1)	5	18	23
Absent (0)	10	72	82
Total	15	90	105

To perform the stratified analysis of these data, the database in Stata is prepared as is seen here:

```
. list
     +-------------------------------------+
     | smoker   hpv   oc    subjects |
     |-------------------------------------|
  1. |      0     1    1          75 |
  2. |      0     1    0          20 |
  3. |      0     0    1           5 |
  4. |      0     0    0          80 |
  5. |      1     1    1           5 |
     |-------------------------------------|
  6. |      1     1    0          18 |
  7. |      1     0    1          10 |
  8. |      1     0    0          72 |
     +-------------------------------------+
```

Using the Mantel–Haenszel method, the following command can be employed to perform the stratified analysis in a case-control study:

```
cc oc hpv [fw=subjects], by(smoker)
```

Output

```
         smoker |       OR        [95% Conf. Interval]   M-H Weight
----------------+------------------------------------------------------
              0 |       60        20.21104   207.9978     .5555556 (exact)
              1 |        2         .4721323  7.399327     1.714286 (exact)
----------------+------------------------------------------------------
          Crude |   21.33333      10.63312   43.91911              (exact)
   M-H combined |   16.1958        8.529819  30.75142
----------------------------------------------------------------------
Test of homogeneity (M-H)    chi2(1) = 18.06    Pr>chi2 = 0.0000

                  Test that combined OR = 1:
                            Mantel-Haenszel chi2(1) = 89.05
                                        Pr>chi2 = 0.0000
```

The output reports the point estimation of the OR for each stratum as well as the crude OR and the weighted OR (M–H combined) with 95% confidence intervals, respectively. In addition, the weighted factor in each stratum is reported (M–H weight) as well as two significance tests. The purposes of these tests are as follows:

1. To assess whether the ORs in all strata are equal: *test of homogeneity* ($H_0 : OR_1 = OR_2 = \cdots = OR_k$).
2. To assess whether the weighted OR is equal to 1: *test of combined* OR $= 1$ ($H_0 : OR_{M-H} = 1$).

The results indicate that there is a significant difference in the ORs of each stratum (*P*-value $< .05$); therefore, it is recommended that the OR be analyzed per stratum. When we compare the point estimates of the OR_0 (60) in nonsmokers and those of the OR_1 (2) in smokers, we can see that the smoking habit modifies the magnitude of the association between HPV and OC. Finally, the estimated magnitude of the association of interest among smokers is 60 (95% CI: 20.2, 207.9), which is statistically significant (*P*-value $< .05$).

7.4 Sample Size and Statistical Power

To determine the minimum sample size for assessing the null hypothesis, H_0: OR = 1, with enough statistical power (i.e., $1 - \beta = 0.8$) and a minimum level of significance (i.e., $\alpha = 0.05$), the classical formula for comparing two proportions is recommended (Rosner, 2010). In Stata, this can be performed in the option that features the chi-squared test comparing two independent proportions with the *Power and sample size analysis* window in the *Statistics* menu (Figure 7.1).

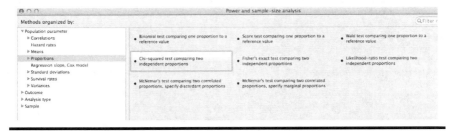

Figure 7.1   Sample size for comparing two independent proportions.

For example (using the data of nonsmokers), to assess the magnitude of the association between HPV status and OC with ORs = 2, 2.5, and 3, assuming that the prevalence estimates of OC in HPV-negatives are 0.10, 0.15, and 0.2, the table of sample size should be filled in for a one-sided test and equal allocation, as illustrated in Figure 7.2.

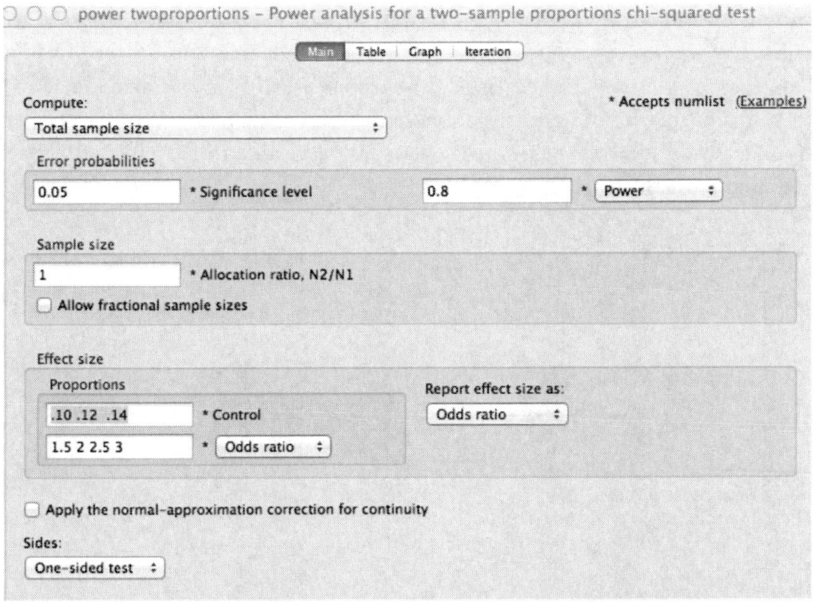

Figure 7.2   Sample size specifications for comparing two independent proportions under different conditions.

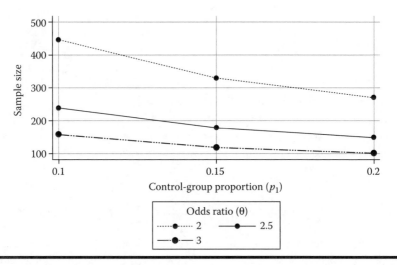

Figure 7.3   Alternatives of sample size for comparing two independent proportions under different conditions. Parameters: α = 0.05, 1 − β = 0.8.

Once the window for the previous requested sample size is submitted with the graph option, a plot is displayed (Figure 7.3). The results show that the lower the OR, the total sample size increases; however, when the proportion of OC in HPV-negative groups is incremented, the differences in sample size are reduced. To determine the sample size for the overall OR while controlling for potential confounders, an adjustment has to be made, as explained in Chapter 8 (Hosmer and Lemeshow, 2000).

Chapter 8

Logistic Regression Model

Aim: Upon completing the chapter, the learner should be able to use a logistic regression model to estimate the magnitude of the association between exposure and disease, controlling for potential confounders.

8.1 Model Definition

The *logistic regression model* is a statistical model that can explain the behavior of a dichotomous variable or a binomial proportion through different predictor variables. In epidemiology these predictors may include variables of exposure, potential confounding variables, and other types of controlling variables. A simple binary logistic regression model (Hosmer and Lemeshow, 2000; Collett, 2002) is defined using the following expression:

$$\Pr(Y_i = 1) = p_i = \frac{e^{-(\beta_0 + \beta_1 X)}}{1 + e^{-(\beta_0 + \beta_1 X)}} = \frac{1}{1 + e^{-(\beta_0 + \beta_1 X)}}$$

where:
p_i indicates the probability of having the diagnosis of interest in the ith subject, that is, the probability of the ith subject being a case
Y indicates a dichotomous variable, coded as $Y = 1$ for a case and $Y = 0$ for a control
X indicates a predictor variable
β_0 indicates the coefficient that is not affected by any predictor
β_1 indicates the coefficient that affects the predictor X

By using the logarithmic transformation of $\left[p_i / (1 - p_i) \right]$, we obtain the *logit* function, as can be seen in the following:

$$g(x) = \text{logit}(p_i) = \ln\left[\frac{p_i}{1 - p_i} \right] = \beta_0 + \beta_1 x$$

where:

β_0 indicates the value of the logit(p_i) when $X = 0$

β_1 indicates changes in the logit(p_i) per unit of change in X

8.2 Parameter Estimation

The logistic regression model is adjusted by estimating the unknown parameters β_0 and β_1. One of the procedures for estimating the unknown parameters is known as the *maximum-likelihood estimation* (MLE), which is based on the likelihood function. This function is given by the joint probability of observing the sample data and is demonstrated in the following:

$$L = \Pr(Y_1, Y_2, \ldots, Y_n)$$

where n is the number of observations or the sample size. The likelihood function provides support for a particular value of the parameter β_i, given an observed data. If the observed data provide more support for one value of the parameter than for another value, then the likelihood is higher for the former parameter value (Marschener, 2015).

Under the assumption that the observed data are independent, the likelihood function can be expressed as follows:

$$L = \Pr(Y_1) * \Pr(Y_2) *, \ldots, * \Pr(Y_n)$$

Defining $\Pr(Y_i)$ depends on the probability distribution of the random variable, Y_i. In the case of binomial distribution, when Y is the binomial proportion in K groups, the likelihood function is defined as

$$L(\beta) = \prod_{i=1}^{K} C_{y_i}^{n_i} * p_i^{y_i} * (1 - p_i)^{n_i - y_i}$$

where:

$C_{y_i}^{n_i}$ is the total number of combinations with y cases given n subjects in the ith group

p_i is the probability of the disease in the ith group

If Y is a dichotomous variable ($Y = 0, 1$), the likelihood function is defined as follows:

$$L(\beta) = \prod_{i=1}^{n} p_i^{y_i} * (1 - p_i)^{1 - y_i}$$

where:

p_i is the probability of having the disease in the ith subject
n is the total number of subjects

In the case of the logistic regression model, we use the coefficients βs that produce the highest value of the likelihood function. The βs obtained in this maximization process are identified as the maximum-likelihood estimates (Hardin and Hilbe, 2001).

8.3 Programming the Logistic Regression Model

There are several commands in Stata that can be used to estimate the parameters of the logistic regression model, including *logit, logistic, binreg,* and *glm.* For example, perhaps the user is interested in exploring the statistical relationship between smoking habits and oral cavity cancer with the following data (Fu et al., 2013):

	Cancer		
Smoker	No (0)	Yes (1)	Total
No (0)	511	333	844
Yes (1)	346	340	686
Total	857	673	1530

Note: Codes of the categories of each variable are shown in parentheses.

The database in Stata is the following:

```
+-------------------------------+
| smoker    cancer    subjects  |
| ----------------------------- |
|    0         0          511   |
|    1         0          346   |
|    0         1          333   |
|    1         1          340   |
+-------------------------------+
```

The estimate of the simple logistic regression model parameters for the above grouped data can be accomplished with different commands. The difference between them is the default output provided and the method used to maximize the likelihood function for parameters' estimation. Some of these commands and their outputs are shown below.

8.3.1 Using glm

```
glm cancer smoker [fw=subjects], fam(bin)
```

Output

```
Generalized linear models             No. of obs      =       1530
Optimization      : ML                Residual df     =       1528
                                      Scale parameter =          1
Deviance          =   2083.154244     (1/df) Deviance = 1.363321
Pearson           =   1529.999986     (1/df) Pearson  = 1.001309

Variance function : V(u) = u*(1-u)      [Bernoulli]
Link function     : g(u) = ln(u/(1-u)) [Logit]

                                      AIC             =     1.364153
Log likelihood    = -1041.577122      BIC             =   -9121.705
------------------------------------------------------------------------
             |               OIM
cancer |    Coef.    Std. Err.    z    P>|z|   [95% Conf. Interval]
--------+---------------------------------------------------------------
Smoker |  0.4107339 0.1038812   3.95  0.000   0.2071305   0.6143372
 _cons |  -0.428227 0.0704269  -6.08  0.000  -0.5662612  -0.2901928
------------------------------------------------------------------------
```

The command *fam(bin)* is used to ensure that the probability distribution of the dependent variable (cancer) will follow a binomial distribution.

8.3.2 Using logit

```
logit cancer smoker [fw=subjects]
```

Output

```
Logistic regression                   Number of obs   =       1530
                                      LR chi2(1)      =      15.69
                                      Prob > chi2     =     0.0001
Log likelihood = -1041.5771           Pseudo R2       =     0.0075


------------------------------------------------------------------------
cancer |    Coef.    Std. Err.    z    P>|z|   [95% Conf. Interval]
--------+---------------------------------------------------------------
smoker |  0.4107339 0.1038812   3.95  0.000   0.2071306   0.6143373
 _cons | -0.4282271 0.0704269  -6.08  0.000  -0.5662613  -0.2901929
------------------------------------------------------------------------
```

8.3.3 Using logistic

```
logistic cancer smoker [fw=subjects], coef
```

Output

```
Logistic regression                      Number of obs    =        1530
                                         LR chi2(1)       =       15.69
                                         Prob > chi2      =      0.0001
Log likelihood = -1041.5771              Pseudo R2        =      0.0075

-----------------------------------------------------------------------
  cancer |    Coef.   Std. Err.    z    P>|z|   [95% Conf.  Interval]
---------+-------------------------------------------------------------
  smoker |  0.4107339 0.1038812   3.95  0.000   0.2071306   0.6143373
   _cons | -0.4282271 0.0704269  -6.08  0.000  -0.5662613  -0.2901929
-----------------------------------------------------------------------
```

To display the estimates of the beta parameters, the **coef** option is used.

8.3.4 Using binreg

```
binreg cancer smoker [fw=subjects], coef ml
```

Output

```
Generalized linear models                No. of obs       =        530
Optimization       : ML                  Residual df      =       1528
                                         Scale parameter  =          1
Deviance        = 2083.154244            (1/df) Deviance  =   1.363321
Pearson         = 1529.999986            (1/df) Pearson   =   1.001309

Variance function: V(u) = u*(1-u)        [Bernoulli]
Link function    : g(u) = ln(u/(1-u))    [Logit]

                                         AIC              =   1.364153
Log likelihood   = -1041.577122          BIC              = -9121.705

-----------------------------------------------------------------------
         |                OIM
  cancer |    Coef.    Std. Err.    z    P>|z|   [95% Conf.  Interval]
---------+-------------------------------------------------------------
  smoker |  0.4107339  0.1038812   3.95  0.000   0.2071305   0.6143372
   _cons | -0.428227   0.0704269  -6.08  0.000  -0.5662612  -0.2901928
-----------------------------------------------------------------------
```

The **coef** option is used to display the estimates of the beta parameters. The option *ml* is for obtaining the maximum-likelihood estimates.

Therefore, the fitted model for all the commands of the simple logistic regression can be determined with the following equation:

$$\text{logit}(p) = -0.43 + 0.41 * \text{smoker}$$

8.4 Alternative Database

A logistic regression model can also be used when the data are summarized as a binomial proportion (number of cases with a characteristic of interest over the number of observations). For example, let us assume the previous example with the following format:

Smoker	Cancer	Total
No (0)	333	844
Yes (1)	340	686

In parentheses are the codes for the smoker categories.

In this case, the database is entered in Stata as follows:

```
. list
     +------------------------+
     | smoker    cases   total |
     |------------------------|
     |    0       333     844 |
     |    1       340     686 |
     +------------------------+
```

The syntax using the *glm* command, under this database structure, is the following:

```
glm cases smoker, fam(bin total)
```

Output

```
Generalized linear models              No. of obs      =          2
Optimization      : ML                 Residual df     =          0
                                       Scale parameter =          1
Deviance       =  7.90479e-14          (1/df) Deviance =          .
Pearson        =  1.60265e-29          (1/df) Pearson  =          .

Variance function: V(u) = u*(1-u/total)   [Binomial]
Link function    : g(u) = ln(u/(total-u)) [Logit]

                                       AIC             =   9.063989
Log likelihood   = -7.063989303        BIC             =   7.90e-14
```

```
---------------------------------------------------------------------
             |                 OIM
       cases |    Coef.    Std. Err.     z     P>|z|   [95% Conf. Interval]
-------------+-------------------------------------------------------
      smoker |  0.4107339  0.1038812   3.95   0.000   0.2071306   0.6143373
       _cons | -0.4282271  0.0704269  -6.08   0.000  -0.5662613  -0.2901929
---------------------------------------------------------------------
```

The **fam(bin)** option is modified to **fam(bin total)** because the dependent variable denotes the number of cases and not the presence or absence of disease (dichotomous scenario).

Similar results can be obtained with the *binreg* command if the following specifications are used:

```
binreg cases smoker, or n(total) ml
```

The *or* and *ml* options are added to estimate the *odds ratio* (OR) using the maximum likelihood method.

8.5 Estimating the Odds Ratio

One of the important applications of the logistic regression model is estimating the strength or magnitude of association between the disease and exposure under study. This model can be expressed as follows:

$$odds_i = \frac{p_i}{1-p_i} = \frac{\left[1/\left(1+e^{-(\beta_0+\beta_1 X)}\right)\right]}{\left\{1-\left[1/\left(1+e^{-(\beta_0+\beta_1 X)}\right)\right]\right\}} = e^{\beta_0+\beta_1 X}$$

Using this expression, the user can obtain the OR. For example, if we assume that X takes 0 for unexposed subjects and 1 for exposed subjects, the resulting OR will be

$$OR_{exp\ vs.unexp} = \frac{odds_{exposed}}{odds_{unexposed}} = \frac{e^{\beta_0+\beta_1}}{e^{\beta_0}} = e^{\beta_1}$$

In this case, the OR is the exponential of the regression coefficient associated with the exposure. The syntax in Stata to estimate the OR of the previous example (using the *glm* command) is as follows:

```
glm cases smoker, fam(bin total) ef nolog noheader
```

Output

```
---------------------------------------------------------------------
            |                OIM
cases       | Odds Ratio   Std. Err.     z    P>|z|   [95% Conf. Interval]
------------+--------------------------------------------------------
smoker      |  1.507924    0.1566449   3.95   0.000   1.230143    1.848431
_cons       |  0.6516634   0.0458946  -6.08   0.000   0.5676437   0.7481193
---------------------------------------------------------------------
```

The *ef* option is added to obtain the estimated OR. The terms **nolog** and **noheader** are used to display only the parameters of the model.

The result indicates that the odds of having oral cavity cancer among smokers is 1.51 (95% CI: 1.23, 1.85) times the odds of having oral cavity cancer among nonsmokers. This OR is known as the crude OR, because the model includes only the exposure variable.

8.6 Significance Tests

8.6.1 Likelihood Ratio Test

Hypothesis testing can be performed for the logistic regression model using the statistic known as *Deviance* (*D*), which is a measure of discrepancy between observed and fitted data. This measure is defined based on the relative comparison of two likelihood functions, as follows (McCullagh and Nelder, 1999):

$$D = -2*\ln\left(\frac{\text{likelihood function} - \text{current model}}{\text{likelihood function} - \text{best model}}\right)$$

where:

likelihood function–current model is calculated with the estimate of the parameter *p* of the binomial distribution using the current logistic model

likelihood function–best model is calculated with the binomial proportion using the observed data

For logistic regression, the equation for *D* is the following:

$$D = -2\sum_{i=1}^{n} y_i \ln\left(\frac{\hat{p}_i}{y_i}\right) + (1 - y_i)\ln\left(\frac{1 - \hat{p}_i}{1 - y_i}\right)$$

This comparison is known as the *likelihood ratio test*. The syntaxes in Stata to perform this test (with the previous database) to assess the effect of the predictor *smoker* are as follows:

```
. quietly: glm cases smoker, fam(bin total)
. estimates store modell
. quietly: glm cases, fam(bin total)
. lrtest modell .
Likelihood-ratio test                    LR chi2(1)   =    15.69
(Assumption: . nested in modell)         Prob > chi2  =    0.0001
```

The results show that removing the predictor *smoker* from the model has a significant effect (*P*-value = .0001). Therefore, it is suggested that it not be removed from the model.

8.6.2 Wald Test

The statistical assessment of specific parameters in the logistic regression model can be performed with the likelihood ratio test. Another option is the Wald test for assessing individual parameters (H_0: $\beta j = 0$) using the following statistic:

$$Z_0 = \frac{\hat{\beta}_j}{SE(\hat{\beta}_j)}$$

where $SE(\hat{\beta}_j)$ is the asymptotic (i.e., large-sample) standard error of $\hat{\beta}_j$. The test statistic Z_0 follows an asymptotic standard-normal distribution, $N(0,1)$, under the null hypothesis.

An equivalent process is to calculate the square of Z_0 and use the chi-squared distribution (χ^2) to assess the null hypothesis, H_0: $\beta_j = 0$. The use of χ^2 is recommended for *two-sided alternatives* $(H_a: \beta_i \neq 0)$. For *one-sided alternatives* $(H_a: \beta_i < 0, H_a: \beta_i > 0)$, the normal distribution is recommended.

The output of the *glm* command for the logistic model shows the Wald test for each predictor. Another Stata command that can be used to perform the Wald test is **test**. For example, using the previous database to assess the effect of the predictor *smoker,* the syntaxes are as follows:

```
glm cases smoker, fam(bin total)
test smoker
```

Output

```
. quietly: glm cases smoker, fam(bin total)
. test smoker
( 1)   [cases]smoker = 0
          chi2( 1) =     15.63
        Prob > chi2 =    0.0001
```

The likelihood ratio test and the Wald test showed the significant effect of the predictor *smoker* in the logistic regression model (P-value = .0001); however, the test statistics differ (15.69 vs. 15.63).

8.7 Extension of the Logistic Regression Model

The logistic regression model can be extended to include as predictors of the potential confounders and the interaction terms formed by the product of the exposure and confounders. When more than one predictor is included, the model is called a *multivariable logistic regression model* and is expressed as follows:

$$Pr(Y_i = 1) = p_i = \frac{1}{1+e^{-\left(\beta_0 + \beta_E * E_i + \Sigma\beta_i C_i + \Sigma\gamma_{(j)i} * (E*C)_{(j)i}\right)}}$$

where:

p_i indicates the probability of the ith subject's having the disease of interest

E indicates the exposure

C_i indicates the ith potential confounding variable

γ_j indicates the jth coefficient or the interaction terms associated with the product of the exposure and the potential confounding variables $(E*C)$

These interaction terms are useful to estimate the magnitude of the association in different strata.

By way of illustration, let us continue to use the previous example, in which the predictor *sex* was included as a potential confounding variable, with the following data distribution:

Smoker	Sex	Cases of Cancer	Total
No (0)	Female (0)	218	477
	Male (1)	115	367
Yes (1)	Female (0)	20	42
	Male (1)	370	694

Note: In parentheses are the codes for the categories of the variables *smoker* and *sex*.

To analyze these data, the following database is created in the Stata data editor:

```
+------------------------------+
| smoker    sex    cases   total |
|------------------------------|
1. |    0      0      218     477 |
2. |    0      1      115     367 |
3. |    1      0       20      42 |
4. |    1      1      370     694 |
+------------------------------+
```

In Stata, the *glm* command can be used in conjunction with the previous database to fit a logistic regression model with interaction terms. The syntax for doing so is as follows:

`xi: glm cases i.smoker*i.sex, fam (bin total) nolog noheader`

Output

```
. xi: glm cases i.smoker*i.sex, fam (bin total) nolog noheader
-----------------------------------------------------------------------
                |              OIM
          cases| Coef.    Std. Err.    z    P>|z|   [95% Conf. Interval]
----------------+------------------------------------------------------
      _Ismoker_1| .0770228  .3223394  0.24  0.811   -.5547508   .7087965
        _Isex_1| -.612164  .1452999 -4.21  0.000   -.8969466  -.3273814
_IsmoXsex_1_1| .8402336  .3497938  2.40  0.016    .1546503  1.525817
          _cons| -.172333  .0919139 -1.87  0.061   -.3524809   .0078149
-----------------------------------------------------------------------
```

The multivariate logistic regression model is determined with the following equation:

$$\text{logit}(p) = -0.17 + 0.08 * \_Ismoker\_1 - 0.6 * \_Isex\_1 + 0.84 * \_IsmoXsex\_1\_1$$

where:

    _Ismoker_1 is a dummy variable with value 1 if the subject smokes, otherwise is 0
    _Isex_1 is a dummy variable with value 1 for males, otherwise is 0
    _IsmoXsex_1_1 is a dummy variable with value 1 if the subject smokes and is a
        male, otherwise is 0

Start the command with **xi:** in the *glm* command to indicate that some of the predictors are defined as categorical. This instruction, when placed prior to the *glm* command, enables us to define the model with interaction terms. The instruction **i.smoker*i.sex** indicates that the logistic regression model will use as predictors *smoker, sex,* and the interaction term formed by the product of these predictors. This form is useful when there are more than two categories in the predictor variables that are defined as being categorical.

In the previous output table, the Wald test shows that there is evidence that the interaction term **_IsmoXsex_1_1** affects the logit(*p*) estimate (*P*-value = .016). An alternative procedure for making a statistical assessment of the interaction term is the likelihood ratio test (*lrtest*), which is recommended when the user is interested in assessing simultaneously several interaction terms. The following commands sequence perform the *lrtest* with the previous database:

```
. quietly xi: glm cases i.smoker*i.sex, fam(bin total)
. estimates store model1
. quietly: glm cases i.smoker, fam(bin total)
lrtest model1 .
Likelihood-ratio test                    LR chi2(2)  =      18.62
(Assumption: . nested in model1)         Prob > chi2 =     0.0001
```

The results indicate that the interaction term composed of *smoker* and *sex* is statistically significant (*P*-value = .0001), which is similar to what was found using the Wald test. Therefore, the variable sex modifies the relationship between smoking status and cancer. As a consequence, it is recommended to estimate sex-specific OR using the *lincom* command as follows:

```
quietly xi: glm cases i.smoker*i.sex, fam(bin total)
*In females
. lincom _Ismoker_1 , or
(1)   [cases]_Ismoker_1 = 0
```

cases	Odds Ratio	Std. Err.	z	P>|z|	[95% Conf. Interval]
(1)	1.080067	.3481481	0.24	0.811	.5742153 2.031545

In females the result indicates that the odds of having oral cavity cancer among smokers is 1.08 (95% CI: 0.57, 2.03) times the odds of having oral cavity cancer among nonsmokers. However, this excess was not statistically significant (*P*-value > .1).

```
*In males

. lincom _Ismoker_1 + _IsmoXsex_1_1, or

( 1)   [cases]_Ismoker_1 + [cases]_IsmoXsex_1_1 = 0

------------------------------------------------------------------------
   cases | Odds Ratio   Std. Err.    z    P>|z|     [95% Conf. Interval]
---------+--------------------------------------------------------------
     (1) |   2.502415    .3399329   6.75   0.000     1.917479    3.26579
------------------------------------------------------------------------
```

In males the result indicates that the odds of having oral cavity cancer among smokers is 2.5 (95% CI: 1.92, 3.27) times the odds of having oral cavity cancer among nonsmokers. This excess was statistically significant (*P*-value < .05).

8.8 Adjusted OR and the Confounding Effect

The logistic regression model without interaction terms allows us to estimate the OR of the exposure of interest, while simultaneously adjusting for potential confounders. Let us assume the following expression of the logistic regression model without interaction terms:

$$\text{Odds} = \frac{p}{1-p} = e^{\beta_0 + \beta_E * E_i + \Sigma \beta_i C_i}$$

If we assume that E is a dichotomous exposure of interest with two categories (0 indicates the absence of exposure and 1 indicates the presence of exposure) and that C_i is a potential confounding variable, then the adjusted OR is obtained following the steps described below:

1. Calculate the odds when the exposure is absent ($E = 0$):

$$\text{Odds}_0 = \frac{p_0}{1-p_0} = e^{\beta_0 + \Sigma \beta_i * C_i'}$$

   where:
   C' is used to distinguish the value of the potential confounders
2. Calculate the odds when the exposure is present ($E_1 = 1$):

$$\text{Odds}_1 = \frac{p_1}{1-p_1} = e^{\beta_0 + \beta_E + \Sigma \beta_i * C_i}$$

3. Calculate the ratio of the odds obtained in steps (1) and (2):

$$OR = \frac{Odds_1}{Odds_0} = e^{\beta_E + \beta_2\left(C_1 - C_1^*\right) + \cdots + \beta_p\left(C_p - C_p^*\right)}$$

When $(C_i - C_i') = 0$, that is, when we assume that the values of the potential confounding variables are equal in exposed and nonexposed subjects, we can obtain the adjusted *odds ratio* ($OR_{adjusted}$), as follows:

$$OR_{adjusted} = e^{\beta_E}$$

The syntax in Stata for obtaining the adjusted odds ratio using the previous data is as follows:

```
xi: glm cases i.smoker i.sex, fam (bin total) ef nolog noheader
```

Output

```
            |                 OIM
      cases | Odds Ratio   Std. Err.     z    P>|z|   [95% Conf. Interval]
------------+----------------------------------------------------------------
  _Ismoker_1 |  2.211517    0.2757527   6.37   0.000    1.732026    2.823749
    _Isex_1 |  0.6247632   0.0825355  -3.56   0.000    0.482243    0.8094034
      _cons |  0.7947862   0.0708192  -2.58   0.010    0.6674276   0.9464473
```

The results indicate that the odds of having oral cavity cancer in smokers is 2.21 (95% CI: 1.73, 2.82) times the odds of having oral cavity cancer in nonsmokers, after adjusting for sex. The difference between the point estimate of the adjusted OR ($\widehat{OR}_{adjusted} = 2.21$) and the point estimate of the crude OR ($\widehat{OR}_{crude} = 1.51$) indicates that the magnitude of association given by the crude OR is underestimated. Therefore, the variable *sex* confounds the relationship between the smoking habit and oral cavity cancer.

8.9 Effect Modification

When the magnitude of the association between the exposure and the disease is explored in different strata, the user can identify effect modification. If the ORs change between strata, using a subjective assessment, then it is expected that the interaction terms in the model will be statistically significant. For example, using the previous example, if we stratify by sex, the point estimates of the ORs are very different ($\widehat{OR}_{smk+vs\ smk-}^{sex=1} = 2.50$ vs. $\widehat{OR}_{smk+vs\ smk-}^{sex=0} = 1.08$), as can be seen in the following results:

```
. xi: glm cases i.smoker if sex==1, fam (bin total) ef nolog noheader
-------------------------------------------------------------------------
           |                OIM
    cases  | Odds Ratio  Std. Err.    z    P>|z|   [95% Conf.  Interval]
-----------+-------------------------------------------------------------
_Ismoker_1 |   2.502415  0.3399329   6.75  0.000    1.917479    3.26579
      _cons|  0.4563492  0.0513548  -6.97  0.000    0.3660228   0.5689662
-------------------------------------------------------------------------

. xi: glm cases i.smoker if sex==0, fam (bin total) ef nolog noheader

-------------------------------------------------------------------------
           |                OIM
    cases  | Odds Ratio  Std. Err.    z    P>|z|   [95% Conf.  Interval]
-----------+-------------------------------------------------------------
_Ismoker_1 |   1.080067  0.3481481   0.24  0.811    0.5742153   2.031545
      _cons|  0.8416988  0.0773638  -1.87  0.061    0.702942    1.007845
-------------------------------------------------------------------------
```

This result indicates that the predictor *sex* has a modifying effect on the relationship between the smoking habit and oral cavity cancer, as was expected (because of the significant results in the *likelihood ratio test*).

8.10 Prevalence Ratio

Several epidemiological studies use the prevalence ratio (PR) to assess the magnitude of the association between exposure and disease. The main reason is that the OR can augment this magnitude, particularly when the prevalence of the outcome among exposure and nonexposure groups is large. To estimate the PR using the logistic regression model, the user needs to use the command *link(log)*. For example, to estimate the PR by sex, the syntax is as follows:

```
glm cases i.smoker if sex==1, fam(bin total) ef link(log)
```

Output

```
-------------------------------------------------------------------------
           |                OIM
    cases  | Risk Ratio  Std. Err.    z    P>|z|    95% Conf.  Interval]
-----------+-------------------------------------------------------------
1.smoker   |   1.701416  0.1446968   6.25  0.000    1.440191    2.010022
      _cons|  0.3133515  0.0242131 -15.02  0.000    0.2693136   0.3645904
-------------------------------------------------------------------------
glm cases i.smoker if sex==0, fam(bin total) ef link(log)
```

Output

```
-------------------------------------------------------------------------
           |                OIM
    cases  | Risk Ratio  Std. Err.    z    P>|z|   [95% Conf.  Interval]
-----------+-------------------------------------------------------------
1.smoker   |    1.04194  0.1764579   0.24  0.808    0.7476307   1.452105
      _cons|  0.4570231  0.0228087 -15.69  0.000    0.4144356   0.5039868
-------------------------------------------------------------------------
```

Among males we can see that there is a substantial difference between the ORs and the PRs; the estimated OR is 2.50 and the estimated PR is 1.70.

Another command that can be used to obtain the PR by sex in a logistic regression model is *binreg*, as follows:

```
binreg cases smoker if sex==1, n(total) rr nolog
```

Output

cases	Risk Ratio	EIM Std. Err.	z	P>|z|	[95% Conf.	Interval]
smoker	1.701416	0.1446966	6.25	0.00	1.440191	2.010022
_cons	0.3133515	0.0242131	-15.02	0.000	0.2693137	0.3645904

```
binreg cases smoker if sex==0, n(total) rr nolog
```

Output

cases	Risk Ratio	EIM Std. Err.	z	P>|z|	[95% Conf.	Interval]
smoker	1.04194	0.1764578	0.24	0.808	0.7476309	1.452105
_cons	0.4570231	0.0228087	-15.69	0.000	0.4144356	0.5039868

The observed results (using binreg and glm), by sex, show that the estimates of the PRs are the same; only slight differences are observed in the standard errors, and these are due to the default methods used to estimate the variance; the *glm* command uses the *maximum-likelihood method,* and *binreg* uses *Fisher's scoring method* (Hardin and Hilbe, 2001; Collett, 2002).

8.11 Nominal and Ordinal Outcomes

The logistic regression model can be extended to handle polytomous outcome (i.e., more than two nominal or ordinal categories). An example of a nominal outcome in an epidemiological case-control study might be a situation in which we have cases (diseased) and two types of controls, which, for example, could be subjects with another disease (control I) and healthy subjects (control II). An example of an ordinal outcome in an epidemiological case-control study might be a situation in which cases (diseased) are categorized by their level of disease severity (e.g., high, moderate, low). In Stata, the programming for these situations can be done with the following commands: *mlogit, ologit,* and *gologit2.*

The logistic regression model in the case of a nominal outcome with more than two categories is called a *multinomial logistic regression model* or *polytomous logistic regression model.* When the outcome is ordinal, the model is called an *ordinal logistic regression model* (Kleinbaum and Klein, 2002). The mathematical expression of both models is based on the ratio of two probabilities defined according to the codes used in the outcome *Y*. For example, assuming *Y* has *k* categories (0, 1, 2, ..., *k*), then the most simple expression of the multinomial regression model is the following:

$$\ln\left(\frac{\Pr[Y=k|E]}{\Pr[Y=0|E]}\right) = \beta_0 + \beta_E * E_{ii}$$

The exponential of the estimated exposure coefficient ($\hat{\beta}_E$) will provide the estimated OR between the category with code k and the category with code 0, as follows:

$$\widehat{OR}_{E+vs.E-}^{(k\,vs.0)} = e^{\hat{\beta}_E}$$

The interpretation of this OR is as follows: in reference to category 0, the probability of being in category *k* among the exposure group is $e^{\hat{\beta}_E}$ times this probability among the nonexposure group's being in category *k*. For the following example, let us assume that we are working with a case-control study to assess the relationship between hepatitis C and receiving a blood transfusion (before 1992), using two types of controls (subjects with hepatitis B and healthy subjects), and using, as well, the following data:

Blood Transfusion	Hepatitis		Healthy (1)
	C (3)	B (2)	Healthy (1)
Yes (1)	19	11	14
No (0)	85	63	220

Note: Codes are in parentheses.

The database in Stata for this study should be as seen below:

```
    +-------------------------------+
    |  hep    trans    subjects     |
    |-------------------------------|
1.  |   1       1          14       |
2.  |   1       0         220       |
3.  |   2       1          11       |
4.  |   2       0          63       |
5.  |   3       1          19       |
    |-------------------------------|
6.  |   3       0          85       |
    +-------------------------------+
```

The syntax in Stata to run the multinomial regression model is as follows:

```
mlogit hep trans [fw=subjects], rrr
```

Output

```
Multinomial logistic regression          Number of obs =     412
                                          LR chi2(2)    =   12.86
                                          Prob > chi2   =  0.0016
Log likelihood = -396.16997              Pseudo R2     =  0.0160
```

```
--------------------------------------------------------------------------
      hep |    RRR     Std. Err.    z    P>|z|  [95% Conf. Interval]
----------+---------------------------------------------------------------
1         | (base outcome)
----------+---------------------------------------------------------------
2         |
    trans | 2.743767   1.17296    2.36  0.018   1.187022   6.342139
    _cons | .2863636  .0409194   -8.75  0.000   .2164148   .3789211
----------+---------------------------------------------------------------
3         |
    trans | 3.512603  1.316033    3.35  0.001   1.685457   7.320497
    _cons | .3863636   .049343   -7.45  0.000  .3008072   .4962543
--------------------------------------------------------------------------
```

The above table shows that in reference to the healthy subjects: the likelihood of hepatitis C among the subjects who had had blood transfusion experience before 1992 is 3.51 (95% CI: 1.69, 7.32) times the likelihood of hepatitis C among the subjects who had not had blood transfusion experience before 1992. This excess was statistically significant (*P*-value = .001).

To use as the reference the subjects with hepatitis B instead of the healthy subjects, you need to use the option *baseoutcome,* as is done in the following:

```
mlogit hep trans [fw=subjects], rrr baseoutcome(2)
```

Output

```
---------------------------------------------------------------------------
      hep |      RRR   Std. Err.      z    P>|z|   [95% Conf. Interval]
----------+----------------------------------------------------------------
1         |
    trans | 0.3644624  0.1558076   -2.36  0.018   0.1576755  0.8424443
    _cons |  3.492063  0.4989922    8.75  0.000    2.639072  4.620756
----------+----------------------------------------------------------------
2         | (base outcome)
----------+----------------------------------------------------------------
3         |
    trans |  1.280212   0.529671    0.60  0.550   0.5689947  2.880417
    _cons |  1.349206  0.2243001    1.80  0.072   0.9740238  1.868905
---------------------------------------------------------------------------
```

The table above indicates that in reference to the subjects with hepatitis B, the likelihood of hepatitis C among the subjects who had had blood transfusion experience before 1992 is 1.28 (95% CI: 0.57, 2.88) times the likelihood of hepatitis C among the subjects who had not had blood transfusion experience before 1992. However, this excess was not statistically significant (*P*-value > .1).

For the ordinal logistic regression model, there are different expressions, the use of each depending on the manner in which the categories are compared. When these categories are grouped and the ORs do not depend on the grouping procedure, it is said that the *proportional odds assumption* is met. The most common expression of this model, under this assumption, is as follows:

$$\ln\left(\frac{\Pr[Y \leq k|E]}{\Pr[Y > k | E]}\right) = \beta_0 - \beta_E * E_i$$

This model combines into two groups the categories of the outcome, as follows: those subjects with categories that are less than or equal to k and those with categories that are greater than k. The negative sign in the coefficient of the exposure occurs because of the way Stata programmed this model; therefore, caution has to be taken to interpret the output and the way the codes of the outcome categories are defined. The exponential of the estimated exposure coefficient, $\hat{\beta}_E$, will provide the estimated OR between categories with code $>k$ and categories with code $\leq k$, due to the following relationship:

$$e^{-\beta_E} = \frac{1}{\widehat{OR}_{E+\text{vs.}E-}^{(\leq k \text{ vs.} >k)}}, \text{ then,}$$

$$\widehat{OR}_{E+\text{vs.}E-}^{(>k \text{ vs.} \leq k)} = e^{\hat{\beta}_E}$$

The interpretation of this OR is as follows: the likelihood of being in a category greater than k among the members of the exposure group is $e^{\hat{\beta}_E}$ times the likelihood of being in a category greater than k among the nonexposure group. To improve the interpretation, use high values of the outcome codes for those subjects with worst outcome. For example, assuming a case-control study to assess the relationship between glycohemoglobin and age, let us suppose that glycohemoglobin is categorized into three groups—using tertiles as the cutoff points—as follows:

Q1: ≤ 5.4 (best)
Q2: >5.4 and ≤ 5.9
Q3: >5.9 (worst)

In addition, let's assume that age was categorized into two groups (above and at or below the mean value of the study sample). Using the available data, then, the following table results:

Age (Years)	Glycohemoglobin Group			Total
	Q1 (1)	Q2 (2)	Q3 (3)	
≤ 45 (0)	14	7	3	24
>45 (1)	9	16	14	39
Total	23	23	17	63

Note: Codes are in parentheses.

The structure of the database in Stata is as seen below:

```
     +-----------------------------+
     | glycon3    age    subjects |
     |-----------------------------|
 1.  |      1       0         14  |
 2.  |      1       1          9  |
 3.  |      2       0          7  |
 4.  |      2       1         16  |
 5.  |      3       0          3  |
     |-----------------------------|
 6.  |      3       1         14  |
     +-----------------------------+
```

The ordinal logistic model can be run with the assumption that the OR depends on the cutoff point of the outcome. Therefore, for every cutoff point in the outcome, one OR is estimated. If we assume that the *proportional odds* assumption is fulfilled, then we would expect all ORs to be equal. The syntax in Stata to run the ordinal logistic model without the proportional odds assumption is as follows:

```
gologit2 glycon3 age [fw=subjects], or
```

Output

```
Generalized Ordered Logit Estimates        Number of obs  =       63
                                           LR chi2(2)     =     8.83
                                           Prob > chi2    =   0.0121
Log likelihood = -64.204942                Pseudo R2      =   0.0643
-------------------------------------------------------------------------
glycon3 | Odds Ratio  Std. Err.    z    P>|z|   [95% Conf. Interval]
--------+----------------------------------------------------------------
1       |
    age | 4.666667    2.622787   2.74   0.006   1.550992    14.04119
  _cons | .7142857    .2957424  -0.81   0.416   .3172788    1.608062
--------+----------------------------------------------------------------
2       |
    age |     3.92    2.750659   1.95   0.052   .9908299    15.50862
  _cons | .1428571    .0881733  -3.15   0.002   .0426117    .4789332
-------------------------------------------------------------------------
```

The *gologit2* command has to be downloaded from Internet.

The numbers in the first column of the above table indicate the way the reference categories are defined. For example, the number 1 indicates that Q1 is the reference category, $\widehat{OR}_{>45 \text{vs.} \leq 45}^{(>5.4 \text{vs.} \leq 5.4)}$. The number 2 indicates that Q1 and Q2 are the reference categories, $\widehat{OR}_{>45 \text{vs.} \leq 45}^{(>5.9 \text{vs.} \leq 5.9)}$.

The interpretation of these ORs is as follows:

1. The likelihood of having a glycohemoglobin higher than 5.4 among subjects older than 45 years is 4.67 (95% CI: 1.55, 14.04) times the likelihood of having a glycohemoglobin higher than 5.4 among subjects 45 years old or younger.
2. The likelihood of having a glycohemoglobin higher than 5.9 among subjects older than 45 years is 3.92 (95% CI: 0.99, 15.51) times the likelihood of having a glycohemoglobin higher than 5.9 among subjects 45 years old or younger.

The syntax in Stata to run the ordinal logistic model, assessing the proportional odds assumption, is as follows:

```
gologit2 glycon3 age [fw= subjects], or autofit lrf
```

Output

```
-------------------------------------------------------------------------------
Testing parallel lines assumption using the .05 level of
significance...

Step 1: Constraints for parallel lines imposed for age
  (P Value = 0.8004)
Step 2: All explanatory variables meet the pl assumption

Wald test of parallel lines assumption for the final model:

( 1)   [1]age - [2]age = 0

          chi2(  1) = 0.06
        Prob > chi2 = 0.8004

An insignificant test statistic indicates that the final model
does not violate the proportional odds/ parallel lines
assumption

If you re-estimate this exact same model with gologit2,
instead of autofit you can save time by using the parameter

pl(age)
-------------------------------------------------------------------------------
Generalized Ordered Logit Estimates      Number of obs   =      63
                                          LR chi2(1)      =    8.77
                                          Prob > chi2     = 0.0031
Log likelihood = -64.236022               Pseudo R2       = 0.0639

( 1)   [1]age - [2]age = 0
-------------------------------------------------------------------------------
 glycon3 | Odds Ratio Std. Err.   z   P>|z| [95% Conf. Interval]
---------+---------------------------------------------------------------------
1        |
     age | 4.427933    2.303347  2.86 0.004 1.597417     12.27394
   _cons | .7293552    .2970438 -0.77 0.438 .3283002     1.620343
```

2						
age	4.427933	2.303347	2.86	0.004	1.597417	12.27394
_cons	.1290829	.0626706	-4.22	0.000	.0498431	.334297

The first assessment in *gologit2* with the *autofit lrf* command is used to determine if there is statistical evidence, based on the likelihood ratio test, that the proportional odds assumption has been fulfilled. If this assumption has been fulfilled, the same OR is estimated for all combinations of the outcome. In this example, the output indicates that the model does not violate the proportional odds assumption (P-value = .8004). As a consequence we interpret only one OR, as follows:

Using as the reference category the participants with the low levels of glycohemoglobin, the likelihood of having high levels of glycohemoglobin among subjects older than 45 years is 4.43 (95% CI: 1.60, 12.27) *times* the likelihood of having high levels of glycohemoglobin among subjects 45 years old or younger.

8.12 Overdispersion

When the logistic regression model is run with grouped data (binomial proportion), the relationship between the *deviance* and the degrees of freedom can be useful in determining the model's goodness of fit (McCullagh and Nelder, 1999; Hardin and Hilbe, 2001). *Overdispersion* occurs when data exhibit more variation than expected. *Underdispersion* occurs when data exhibit less variation than expected. Because *deviance* is a random variable with chi-squared distribution, if the model is adequate to explain the binomial proportion, then it is expected that the observed deviance would be close to the degrees of freedom of the model *(equidispersion)*. For example, if we run the model with only the predictor *smoker* in the example of cancer explained by smoker and sex, we discover that the deviance is 18.62, with 2 degrees of freedom; therefore, overdispersion is observed. To assess the departure between the deviance and the degrees of freedom, we can use the P-value to determine the statistical significance of this difference. The syntax to perform this in Stata is as follows:

```
dis chi2tail(2,18.62)
.00009051
```

The results show that there is a significant difference between the deviance and its degrees of freedom (P-value = 0.00009051). Therefore, the logistic regression model using only the predictor *smoker* is not adequate. Either including more predictors or exploring other models would be another option to consider at this point.

8.13 Sample Size and Statistical Power

To determine the total minimum sample size for assessing the adjusted OR in a case-control study with enough statistical power (i.e., $1 - \beta = 0.8$), a minimum significance level (i.e., $\alpha = 0.05$), and using an unconditional multivariable logistic regression model with one exposure and different covariates, the following expression (Hosmer and Lemeshow, 2000) can be used:

$$n = \frac{\left(1+2P_0\right)}{1-\rho^2} * \frac{\left(Z_{1-\alpha}\sqrt{\left(1/1-\pi\right)+\left(1/\pi\right)} + Z_{1-\beta}\sqrt{\left(1/1-\pi\right)+\left(1/\pi e^{\beta_E}\right)}\right)^2}{P_0 * \beta_E^2}$$

where:

$Z_{1-\alpha}$ and Z_β denote the upper α and β percentage points, respectively, of the standard normal distribution

π denotes the fraction of subjects in the study who are not exposed

P_0 denotes the probability of being a case among those who are not exposed

ρ^2 denotes the squared correlation between the observed and fitted values of the exposure (dichotomous variable) using a logistic regression model, as follows: $\text{logit}\left(\text{pr}[E=1]\right) = \beta_0 + \sum \beta_0 * X_i$

This can be used to estimate pseudo R^2, as follows:

$$\text{pseudo } R^2 = 1 - \frac{L_p}{L_0}$$

where:

L_0 and L_p denote the log likelihoods for models containing only the intercept and the model containing the intercept plus the p-covariates, respectively

β_E denotes the coefficient of the exposure in the multivariate logistic regression model for the outcome of interest under the alternative hypothesis. If we assume that OR = 2, then β_E is approximately 0.69314 {ln(2) = 0.69314}

Based on the data presented previously, the purpose of which was to assess the magnitude of the association between cancer and the smoking habit adjusted by sex ($\widehat{OR}_{adj} = 2.21$), the parameters needed to obtain the minimum sample size are as follows:

$$\beta_E = \ln\left(2.21\right) = 0.7929, \Pi = 0.4658, P_0 = 0.3945, \rho^2 = 0.5679,$$

$$Z_{0.95} = 1.96, Z_{0.80} = 1.28$$

Therefore,

$$n = \frac{\left(1+2*.3945\right)}{1-0.5679}$$

$$* \frac{\left(1.96*\sqrt{\left(1/1-0.4658\right)+\left(1/0.4658\right)} + 1.28\sqrt{\left(1/1-0.4658\right)+\left(1/0.4658e^{.7929}\right)}\right)^2}{0.3945*0.7929^2}$$

$$= 618.64$$

It is desirable for the result to be divisible by 2, given that a total sample size of about 619, or 310, per group would be the minimum required. Unfortunately, Stata does not provide the option in its power and sample size calculation tool for this formula. Therefore, a *do-file* has to be programmed with the following sequence of commands (and assuming the data of the previous example):

```
gen a=(1+2*.3945)/(1-.5679)
gen b=1.96*sqrt((1/(1-.4658))+(1/.4658))
gen c=1.28*sqrt( (1/(1-.4658)) + (1/(.4658*exp(.7929))))
gen d=.3945*.7929^2
gen n=a*((b+c)^2)/d
```

Before running these commands, go to *edit* and create a dataset with one variable, such as *id,* and one space row. The other option is to work interactively with Stata by invoking the *mata* command, as follows:

```
. mata
------------------ mata (type end to exit) -----------------
: a=(1+2*.3945)/(1-.5679)
: b=1.96*sqrt((1/(1-.4658))+(1/.4658))
: c=1.28*sqrt( (1/(1-.4658)) + (1/(.4658*exp(.7929))))
: d=.3945*.7929^2
: n=a*((b+c)^2)/d
: n
  618.6378426
: end
------------------------------------------------------------
```

Mata is a matrix programming language that can be used interactively or as an extension for do-files and ado-files. To extend the information about *mata* command, we recommend checking out the book by Baum (*An Introduction to Stata Programming,* 2009).

Chapter 9

Poisson Regression Model

Aim: Upon completing the chapter, the learner should be able to estimate the magnitude of the association between disease and exposure, controlling for potential confounders, using a Poisson regression model.

9.1 Model Definition

The Poisson regression model allows us to assess epidemiological studies when the main outcome is an integer number, such as the number of cancer patients, number of immunized children, or number of hospitalized patients. It is assumed that these types of outcomes, Y, are random variables with positive integers and are distributed as the *Poisson probability distribution*. This probability distribution is characterized by one parameter, identified by the Greek letter μ, which is the expected number of events of the outcome of interest and is expressed in the following manner:

$$\Pr[Y = y] = \frac{e^{-\mu}\mu^{y}}{y!}$$

where the variance of Y is equal to the expected value of Y, $\mathrm{Var}(Y) = E(Y) = \mu$.

The Poisson regression model is used in cohort studies to estimate the expected value of Y among exposure and nonexposure groups, adjusted for the effect of potential confounders. An example of this would be the expected number of lung cancer cases in a 5-year period among smokers and nonsmokers, adjusted for the effects of age and sex (Fox, 2008; Hoffmann, 2004). One advantage of this model is that it can be used to obtain an estimate of the *relative risk (RR)*, adjusted for potential confounders. The simplest form of a Poisson regression model, with an exposure variable (E) and one potential confounding variable (C), can be defined with any of the following equivalent expressions:

$$[\text{i}] \qquad \mu_i = T_i * I_i = T_i * e^{\beta_0 + \beta_E * E + \beta_C * C + \beta_{EC} * (EC)}$$

$$[\text{ii}] \qquad I_i = \mu_i / T_i = e^{\beta_0 + \beta_E * E + \beta_C * C + \beta_{EC} * (EC)}$$

$$[\text{iii}] \quad Ln(\mu_i) = Ln(T_i) + \beta_0 + \beta_E * E + \beta_C * C + \beta_{EC} * (EC)$$

$$[\text{iv}] \quad Ln(I_i) = \beta_0 + \beta_E * E + \beta_C * C + \beta_{EC} * (EC)$$

where:

μ_i indicates the expected value for the outcome variable

I_i represents the incidence (the expected cases by time unit or population under the ith condition)

T_i represents the sum of the times in the study under the ith condition

E denotes the exposure variable

C denotes the effect of the confounder variable

$E*C$ denotes the interaction between the exposure and confounder

β_j denotes the coefficients (parameters) associated with the jth predictor variables ($j = E$, C, or $E * C$); this value represents the expected changes in the natural logarithm of μ_i in the expression [iii]

β_0 represents the constant term (intercept) in the model

The expression $Ln(T_i)$ denotes the natural logarithm of T_i under the expression [iii] of the Poisson regression model, which is included as a predictor variable with a coefficient or parameter equal to 1. This type of predictor is identified as an *offset* and has a fixed parameter.

9.2 Relative Risk

In the event that the outcome variable Y indicates the occurrence of new cases of a disease in a cohort study, we can determine the incidence of this disease among different groups of exposure through a Poisson regression model, as follows (assuming E is dichotomous and C is continuous):

Exposure *(E = 1)*

$$I_{\exp} = \frac{\mu_{\exp}}{T_{\exp}} = e^{\beta_0 + \beta_E + \beta_C * C + \beta_{EC} * C}$$

Nonexposure *(E = 0)*

$$I_{\text{non-exp}} = \frac{\mu_{\text{non-exp}}}{T_{\text{non-exp}}} = e^{\beta_0 + \beta_C * C'}$$

If $C = C'$, then

$$RR = \frac{I_{exp}}{I_{non\text{-}exp}} = e^{\beta_E + \beta_{E \cdot C} * C}$$

In the case of nonsignificant interaction terms (H_0: $\beta_{E*C} = 0$), we can obtain the adjusted RR using the following:

$$RR_{adjusted} = \frac{I_{exp}}{I_{non\text{-}exp}} = e^{\beta_E^*}$$

where β_E^* is obtained from the model that excludes the interaction term. If the interaction term is significant, it is necessary to estimate the RR in different population subgroups defined by the levels of C.

9.3 Parameter Estimation

The procedure for estimating the unknown coefficients in the Poisson regression model is similar to the procedure of logistic regression for obtaining the maximum-likelihood estimates. Under the assumption that the observations are independent, the *likelihood function* for the Poisson regression model is expressed as follows:

$$L(\beta) = \prod_{i=1}^{K} \frac{e^{-\mu_i} \mu_i^y}{y!}$$

where μ_i is the expected value of Y under the ith condition in the Poisson regression model. The coefficients βs that produce the highest value of this likelihood function are the maximum-likelihood estimates (MLEs) for this model. Based on the MLEs estimates, we can also estimate the RRs and test the statistical hypothesis, with the approach similar to that performed for the logistic regression model.

9.4 Example

Suppose we are interested in assessing the difference in the incidence of cardiovascular disease by *sex*, controlling for *age*. Available data for this purpose can be extracted from the epidemiological cohort study of Framingham (Massachusetts), which started in 1948 with a sample of 5,127 subjects, aged 30–62 years old. The following table summarizes the incidence of cardiovascular disease by age and sex:

Age	CVD_M	PY_M	I_M	CVD_F	PY_F	I_F	$RR_{M:F}$
<46	43	7,370	5.83	9	9,205	0.98	5.97
46–55	163	12,649	12.89	71	16,708	4.25	3.03
56–60	155	7,184	21.58	105	10,139	10.36	2.08
61–80	443	15,015	29.50	415	24,338	17.05	1.73
>80	19	470	40.43	50	1,383	36.15	1.12
Total	823	42,688	19.28	650	61,773	10.52	1.83

Note: M, male; F, female; CVD, cardiovascular disease; PY, person-years; and I, incidence per 1,000 persons in 1 year.

The last column of the table shows the RRs between males and females by age group. The observed trend in these RRs indicates that, in the older age groups, the RRs are getting close to 1; therefore, the incidences of cardiovascular disease by sex are quite different for the younger age groups and quite similar for the older age groups. This trend suggests that age has a modifying effect on the relationship between sex and cardiovascular disease (Szklo and Nieto, 2004).

9.5 Programming the Poisson Regression Model

To evaluate the expected number of cases in the Framingham Study by sex and age using the Poisson model, we need to prepare the database as follows:

```
     +-------------------------+
     | age   sex      py   cvd |
     |-------------------------|
 1.  |  1     1     7370    43 |
 2.  |  1     0     9205     9 |
 3.  |  2     1    12649   163 |
 4.  |  2     0    16708    71 |
 5.  |  3     1     7184   155 |
     |-------------------------|
 6.  |  3     0    10139   105 |
 7.  |  4     1    15015   443 |
 8.  |  4     0    24338   415 |
 9.  |  5     1      470    19 |
10.  |  5     0     1383    50 |
     +-------------------------+
```

Note:

- age indicates the code of the age group (1: <46 years; 2: 46–55 years; 3: 56–60 years; 4: 61–80 years; 5: >80 years)
- sex indicates the code of the sex (0 = female, 1 = male)
- py indicates person-years
- cvd indicates the number of cardiovascular disease cases

9.6 Assessing Interaction Terms

According to the trend in the RRs (by age group) that was observed in the previous table, which suggests the presence of an age–sex interaction, we will initially explore the interaction terms in the Poisson regression model using the likelihood ratio test, as follows:

```
. quietly xi: glm cvd i.sex*i.age, fam(poi) lnoff(py)

. estimates store model1

. quietly xi: glm cvd i.sex i.age, fam(poi) lnoff(py)

. lrtest model1 .
```

```
Likelihood-ratio test                  LR chi2(4)   =    29.58
(Assumption: . nested in model1)       Prob > chi2  =   0.0000
```

Note: lnoff(py) indicates the inclusion of the natural logarithm of the py variable as an *offset* variable.

The results indicate a significant age–sex interaction term (*P*-value < .0001), confirming that age has a modifying effect on the relationship that exists between sex and cardiovascular disease. Therefore, it is necessary to estimate the RR (male vs. female) by age group. To carry out this evaluation, we use the Poisson regression model, while also including interaction terms. For example, the resulting models of previous data can be programmed in Stata with the following command:

```
xi: glm cvd i.sex*i.age, fam(poisson) lnoff(py)
```

Output

```
Generalized linear models        No. of obs       =         10
Optimization      : ML           Residual df      =          0
                                 Scale parameter  =          1
Deviance       = 5.31308e-13     (1/df) Deviance  =          .
Pearson        = 4.76108e-13     (1/df) Pearson   =          .

Variance function: V(u) = u          [Poisson]
```

```
Link function      : g(u) = ln(u)        [Log]

                                         AIC         =   8.241062
Log likelihood   = -31.20531135          BIC         =   5.31e-13
```

cvd	Coef.	OIM Std. Err.	z	P>|z|	[95% Conf. Interval]
_Isex_1	1.786304	.3665609	4.87	0.000	1.067858 2.504751
_Iage_2	1.469314	.3538299	4.15	0.000	.7758204 2.162808
_Iage_3	2.360093	.3473253	6.80	0.000	1.679348 3.040838
_Iage_4	2.858762	.3369284	8.48	0.000	2.198394 3.519129
_Iage_5	3.61029	.3620926	9.97	0.000	2.900601 4.319979
_IsexXage_1_2	-.6769246	.3931747	-1.72	0.085	-1.447533 .0936837
_IsexXage_1_3	-1.052307	.38774	-2.71	0.007	-1.812263 -.2923501
_IsexXage_1_4	-1.238024	.3728725	-3.32	0.001	-1.968841 -.5072074
_IsexXage_1_5	-1.674611	.4549709	-3.68	0.000	-2.566337 -.7828843
_cons	-6.930277	.3333333	-20.79	0.000	-7.583599 -6.276956
ln(py)	1	(exposure)			

The resulting equation of the Poisson regression model, using only one decimal approximation of the estimated coefficient of this output, is as follows:

$$Ln\left(\hat{\mu}_i / PY_i\right) = -6.9 + 1.8 * \_Isex\_1 + 1.5 * \_Iage\_2 + 2.4 * \_Iage\_3 + 2.9 * \_Iage\_4$$

$$+ 3.6 * \_Iage\_5 - 0.7 * \_IsexXage\_1\_2 - 1.1 * \_IsexXage\_1\_3$$

$$- 1.2 * \_IsexXage\_1\_4 - 1.7 * \_IsexXage\_1\_5$$

where:

PY_i = person-years

_Isex_1 = 1, if sex = M; _Isex_1 = 0 if sex = F

_Iage_2 = 1, if group of age "2"; _Iage_2 = 0 other groups of age

_Iage_3 = 1, if group of age "3"; _Iage_3 = 0 other groups of age

_Iage_4 = 1, if group of age "4"; _Iage_4 = 0 other groups of age

_Iage_5 = 1, if group of age "5"; _Iage_5 = 0 other groups of age

_IsexXage_1_2 = 1, if _Isex_1 = 1 and _Iage_2 = 1, otherwise 0

_IsexXage_1_3 = 1, if _Isex_1 = 1 and _Iage_3 = 1, otherwise 0

_IsexXage_1_4 = 1, if _Isex_1 = 1 and _Iage_4 = 1, otherwise 0

_IsexXage_1_5 = 1, if _Isex_1 = 1 and _Iage_5 = 1, otherwise 0

Considering the previous estimated coefficients, and using the expression [ii] of the Poisson model, we can determine the age-specific incidences as follows:

1. Incidence for the <46 years age group (age2 = 0, age3 = 0, age4 = 0, age5 = 0):

$$I_{<46} = e^{(-6.9 + 1.8 * \_Isex\_1)}$$

2. Incidence for the 46–55 years age group (age2 = 1, age3 = 0, age4 = 0, age5 = 0):

$$I_{46-55} = e^{(-6.9+1.8*\_Isex\_1+1.5*\_Iage\_2-0.7*\_IsexXage\_1\_2)}$$

3. Incidence for the 56–60 years age group (age2 = 0, age3 = 1, age4 = 0, age5 = 0):

$$I_{56-60} = e^{(-6.9+1.8*\_Isex\_1+2.4*\_Iage\_3-1.1*\_IsexXage\_1\_3)}$$

4. Incidence for the 61–80 years age group (age2 = 0, age3 = 0, age4 = 1, age5 = 0):

$$I_{61-80} = e^{(-6.9+1.8*\_Isex\_1+2.9*\_Iage\_4-1.2*\_IsexXage\_1\_4)}$$

5. Incidence for the >80 years age group (age2 = 0, age3 = 0, age4 = 0, age5 = 1):

$$I_{>80} = e^{(-6.9+1.8*\_Isex\_1+3.6*\_Iage\_5-1.7*\_IsexXage\_1\_5)}$$

Therefore, to estimate the relative risk (males vs. females) for the first two age groups. We estimate the incidence by sex and then divide these incidences in each age group as follows:

1. The <46 years age group:
   When $\_Isex\_1 = 1$,

$$I_{male} = e^{(-6.9+1.8)}$$

   And when $\_Isex\_1 = 0$,

$$I_{female} = e^{(-6.9)}$$

   Then,

$$RR = \frac{I_{male}}{I_{female}} = e^{(1.8)} = 5.96$$

2. The 46–55 years age group:
   When $\_Isex\_1 = 1$ and $\_IsexXage\_1\_2 = 1$,

$$I_{male} = I_{46-55} = e^{(-6.9 + 1.8 + 1.5 - 0.7)}$$

And when $\_Isex\_1 = 0$ and $\_IsexXage\_1\_2 = 1$,

$$I_{\text{female}} = e^{(-6.9+1.5)}$$

Then

$$RR = \frac{I_{\text{male}}}{I_{\text{female}}} = \exp(1.8 - 0.7) = 3.03$$

To facilitate the estimation of these RRs with 95% confidence intervals in Stata, we can use the *lincom* command in the model, with interaction terms, instead of having one model for each age group. To use this command, after running the model with interaction terms, we enter the name of the predictor with the name Stata assigned to it; then we add the plus sign (+) followed by the corresponding interaction terms and the option *irr*. The syntaxes for the first two age groups will be as follows:

For the <46 years age group:

```
xi: glm cvd i.sex*i.age, fam(poisson) lnoff(py)
        lincom _Isex_1, irr
```

Output

```
(1)   [cvd]_Isex_1 = 0
---------------------------------------------------------------------
    cvd |        IRR   Std. Err.    z   P>|z|   [95% Conf. Interval]
--------+------------------------------------------------------------
    (1) |   5.967359    2.1874    4.87  0.000   2.909142    12.24051
---------------------------------------------------------------------
```

The incidence of cardiovascular disease in males younger than 46 years old is 5.97 (95% CI: 2.91, 12.24) times the incidence of cardiovascular disease in females younger than 46 years. This greater level of risk is highly significant (*P*-value < .001).

For the 46–55 years age group:

```
lincom _Isex_1 + _IsexXage_1_2, irr
```

Output

```
(1) [cvd]_Isex_1 + [cvd]_IsexXage_1_2 = 0
---------------------------------------------------------------------
    cvd |        IRR   Std. Err.    z   P>|z|   [95% Conf. Interval]
--------+------------------------------------------------------------
    (1) |  3.032477   .4312037   7.80  0.000   2.294884    4.007138
---------------------------------------------------------------------
```

The incidence of cardiovascular disease in males aged 46–55 years old is 3.03 (95% CI: 2.29, 4.01) times the incidence of cardiovascular disease in females aged 46–55 years old. This greater level of risk is highly significant (*P*-value < .001).

9.7 Overdispersion

Using the Poisson regression model, we can also assess the goodness of fit of the model, as was shown in the previous chapter. For example, if we run the model using only the predictor *sex* (in the previous database) as follows:

```
.  xi: glm cvd i.sex, fam(poi) lnoff(py)
```

```
Generalized linear models             No. of obs      =          10
Optimization         : ML             Residual df     =           8
                                      Scale parameter =           1
Deviance         =   555.0977773      (1/df) Deviance =    69.38722
Pearson          =   517.3470186      (1/df) Pearson  =    64.66838

Variance function: V(u) = u           [Poisson]
Link function    : g(u) = ln(u)       [Log]

                                      AIC             =    62.15084
Log likelihood   =     -308.7542      BIC             =    536.6771
```

```
------------------------------------------------------------------------------
             |               OIM
         cvd |      Coef.   Std. Err.      z    P>|z|    [95% Conf. Interval]
-------------+----------------------------------------------------------------
     _Isex_1 |   .6055324   .0524741    11.54   0.000     .5026851    .7083797
        cons |  -4.554249   .0392232  -116.11   0.000    -4.631125   -4.477373
       ln(py)|          1  (exposure)
------------------------------------------------------------------------------
```

We discover that the deviance is 555.10, with 8 degrees of freedom; therefore, overdispersion is observed. To assess the departure between the deviance and the degrees of freedom, we obtain the *P*-value in Stata, in the following manner:

```
dis chi2tail(8,555.09)
```

```
1.05e-114
```

The results show a very highly significant difference between the deviance and its degrees of freedom (*P*-value < .001). Therefore, the Poisson regression model using only the predictor *sex* is not adequate; including more predictors, exploring another type of model, or assessing the potential correlation between adjacent age groups is called for. For more discussion on this topic, we recommend checking out the books by Cameron and Trivedi (1998), Hilbe (2007), Hoffmann (2004), and Kleinbaum et al. (2008).

Chapter 10

Survival Analysis

Aim: Upon completing the chapter, the learner should be able to use the Cox proportional hazards model to estimate the magnitude of the association between the risk of the occurrence of a given clinical event (e.g., disease, death, remission) after a certain period of time and a factor of exposure, controlling for potential confounders.

10.1 Introduction

In this chapter we present the use of a regression model to analyze the occurrence of an event after a certain time. This analysis is regularly identified as a *survival analysis* or a *time to event analysis* (Kleinbaum and Klein, 2005). The objective in survival analysis is to assess the time it takes for an event of interest to occur when there is the possibility that this event will not occur in all subjects under study. Take the following examples:

Event of Interest	Time of Study	At the End of the Study
Death	Time that a person remains alive after heart surgery until the event of interest occurs.	There are persons who remain alive after heart surgery.
Development of a respiratory disease	Time without developing a respiratory disease after exposure to an environmental contaminant until the event of interest occurs.	There are persons who do not develop a respiratory disease after being exposed to an environmental contaminant.
Hospital discharge after 24 h	Length of hospital stay of a patient who arrives at an emergency room until the event of interest occurs.	There are people who stay in the hospital for longer than 24 h.

For the analysis of survival times, it is necessary to identify a start date for participation in the study. Some possible start dates are date of birth, date of diagnosis, therapy start date, and date or time of an exposure to a toxin. In addition, it is also necessary to identify the date on which the event of interest occurs or the date of study completion.

The study time in survival analysis is determined by the difference between the date of the occurrence of the event of interest and the start date of the study:

$$T = \text{date of occurrence of event under study} - \text{start date}$$

where T can be measured in days, months, years, or some other time unit.

The use of survival analysis is justified when there is a possibility that an event of interest will not occur in a high number of subjects during a given study period, meaning that there will be a high number of individuals with incomplete information. The time of occurrence of the event of interest (T) cannot be exactly determined when the event does not happen; only the minimum survival time (t) (in which the event of interest does not occur in the individual) can be determined. Therefore, the formulation of a study problem in survival analysis with the event's date or time of occurrence being unknown is given by the following expression:

$$T \geq t$$

Censoring information may arise in the following situations:

■ Termination of the research study
■ Loss of follow-up due to the voluntary withdrawal from the study (reasons unrelated to the study)

- Death, assuming that this is not the event of interest
- Development of a disease or health condition that is not associated with the event of interest

When the study time of a subject has not been determined, we use the term censored. If the date of the event's occurrence is unknown, the incomplete data in the survival analysis are called right censoring. The existence of censored observations can be attributed to a selection bias, unless it can be assured that censored individuals are representative of the study population. Therefore, censoring has to be independent of t.

A survival analysis involves a longitudinal design in which there is a recruitment period and a maximum date of observation, as illustrated in the following:

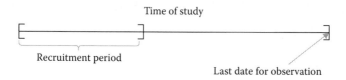

Recruitment time comprises a fixed period of time during which the initial measurement of the study subjects for survival analysis is performed. The maximum date of observation indicates the last day or the specific time to observe the occurrence of an event. The possible situations that may occur while observing the event of interest are illustrated in Figure 10.1.

Situation A. The occurrence of the event after the completion of the study (censored).

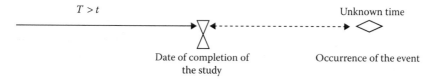

Situation B. The occurrence of the event before the completion of the study.

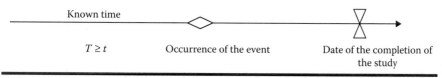

Figure 10.1   Occurrence of the Event in Survival Analysis.

10.2 Probability of Survival

In a survival study, the evaluation $T = t$ cannot be established for censored observations. If there are no censored observations, then the variable T can be analyzed using the standard methods for evaluating a continuous variable (e.g., linear regression, ANOVA). In the case of censored observations, we can ensure only that the event occurred after a time greater than t ($T > t$). For this reason, one of the main objectives in a survival analysis is to determine the probability of $T > t$. This probability is expressed as follows:

$$S(t) = \Pr[T > t]$$

$S(t)$ is defined as the *survival function* and indicates the probability of being free of the event of interest at least at t; that is, the probability of the event occurring after t.

10.3 Components of the Study Design

To perform a survival analysis, the minimum information that must be provided by the study design is: (1) recruitment date, (2) date of the occurrence of the study event, and (3) last date of observation (which could be the date of study termination or the occurrence of the study event). For example, let us assume that the time distribution of seven subjects with cancer in a survival analysis design is as illustrated in Figure 10.2.

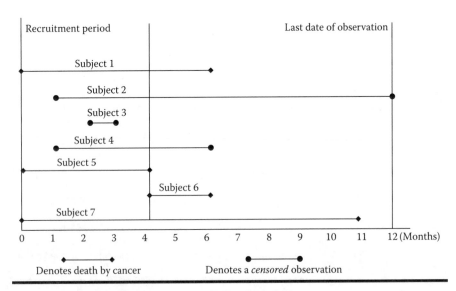

Figure 10.2   Longitudinal design in survival analysis.

In the above illustration, the following patterns occur: (1) the recruitment date is different for every subject; (2) the date of the occurrence of the study event is also different in each subject; (3) the last date of observation is the same for all subjects, 12 months; however, not all the subjects get free of the event at this point. Usually, this type of information can be summarized in the following table:

Subject	Entrance Month	Month of Death or Censored	Death (D) Censored (C)	Survival Time
1	0	6	D	6
2	1	12	C	11
3	2	3	C	1
4	1	6	C	5
5	0	4	D	4
6	4	6	D	2
7	0	11	D	11

When there are censored observations, there are several nonparametric methods for estimating $S(t)$. The life-table estimate of the survivor function, also known as the *actuarial estimate* of survivor function, assumes that the censoring process is such that the censored survival times occur uniformly within different series of time intervals. Another method for estimating the survival function, $S(t)$, is through the Kaplan–Meier (KM) method. This method determines the probability of surviving at least to time $t_{(j)}$. Time $t_{(j)}$ indicates the times at which one or more events have occurred and is sorted in ascending order:

$$t_{(1)} \leq t_{(2)} \leq t_{(3)} \leq \cdots \leq t_{(j-1)} \leq t_{(j)} \leq \cdots$$

where $t_{(1)}$ is the time at which the event of least time occurred.

10.4 Kaplan–Meier Method

To describe the procedure to estimate the survival function of a person, $S(t_{(j)})$, we use the KM method. This method is based on the product of survival function at time $t_{(j-1)}$ and the conditional probability that the event of interest will occur after $t_{(j)}$, given that the person is alive at least until $t_{(j)}$. This product is expressed as follows:

$$S\left(t_{(j)}\right) = S\left(t_{(j-1)}\right) * \Pr\left(T > t_{(j)} \middle| T \geq t_{(j)}\right)$$

where $\Pr[T > t_{(j)} | T \geq t_{(j)}]$ indicates the probability, among those persons who reached $t_{(j)}$ alive, of remaining alive after that specific time,

- $t_{(j)}$ indicates the time in j order in which at least one event occurs after the data are ordered from least to greatest
- $S(t_{(j-1)})$ is the function of survival until time $t_{(j-1)}$

The development of the previous expression with the data from the previous example is presented in the following table:

$T(j)$	r_j^a	f_j^b	$\Pr[T > t_{(j)} | T \geq t_{(j)}]^c$	$S(t_j)$
0	7	0	$1 - (0/7) = 1$	1.0
1^d	–	–	–	–
2	6	1	$1 - (1/6) = 0.833$	0.833
4	5	1	$1 - (1/5) = 0.8$	0.666
5^d	–	–	–	–
6	3	1	$1 - (1/3) = 0.667$	0.44
11^d	–	–	–	–
11	1	1	$1 - (1/1) = 0$	0

[a] r_j indicates the subjects that are at risk an instant before $t_{(j)}$.
[b] f_j indicates the number of deaths in j time.
[c] $\Pr[T > t_{(j)} | T \geq t_{(j)}] = 1 - (f_j/r_j)$.
[d] censored cases.

The $S(t_{(j)})$ usually is graphically represented as a step function; it means that $S(t_{(j)})$ probability remains constant until the time when the next event of interest occurs.

10.5 Programming of $S(t)$

Let us assume a study aimed at assessing oropharyngeal cancer mortality by sex ($1 =$ Males, $2 =$ Females), adjusting for tumor stage (1, 2, and 3). Further, let us suppose that we have the observation time (months) after the diagnosis in 87 subjects, as follows:

id	death	sex	stage	time	id	death	sex	stage	time
1	1	2	2	34	46	0	2	1	28
2	1	2	2	61	47	1	1	2	39
3	0	2	1	78	48	1	1	2	8
4	0	1	2	95	49	1	2	1	35
5	1	2	2	49	50	0	1	1	5
6	1	2	2	59	51	0	1	1	45
7	0	2	2	2	52	1	2	2	0
8	0	2	2	1	53	0	2	2	17
9	1	1	3	6	54	0	2	1	0
10	0	1	1	53	55	0	1	2	1
11	1	2	2	8	56	0	2	1	39
12	0	1	2	21	57	1	2	1	9
13	1	2	3	71	58	1	1	2	5
14	1	1	3	47	59	1	2	2	2
15	0	1	2	35	60	0	1	2	38
16	0	1	1	1	61	1	2	1	41
17	1	2	3	10	62	0	2	2	6
18	0	1	2	7	63	1	2	1	28
19	0	2	2	1	64	0	2	1	60
20	1	1	2	27	65	0	2	2	1
21	0	1	2	34	66	1	2	1	81
22	1	2	3	10	67	0	2	1	2
23	1	2	2	43	68	0	1	1	5
24	0	1	2	84	69	0	1	2	2
25	1	2	2	89	70	0	2	2	44
26	1	2	2	6	71	1	2	3	8

id	death	sex	stage	time	id	death	sex	stage	time
27	0	2	2	4	72	1	1	3	7
28	0	2	2	0	73	0	1	2	5
29	0	2	1	22	74	0	2	2	3
30	1	2	3	1	75	1	2	1	3
31	1	2	1	23	76	1	2	2	2
32	1	2	3	37	77	1	1	2	55
33	1	2	1	25	78	1	2	1	46
34	0	2	1	0	79	0	2	1	70
35	0	2	3	1	80	1	2	1	39
36	1	2	2	39	81	1	1	1	99
37	1	2	1	20	82	0	1	2	5
38	0	1	2	48	83	1	1	2	52
39	1	1	2	20	84	1	2	3	12
40	1	2	2	6	85	0	2	1	39
41	0	2	1	44	86	1	1	1	40
42	1	2	3	13	87	0	1	2	73
43	0	1	3	1					
44	0	2	2	50					
45	0	2	1	0					

To run a survival analysis in Stata, we have to specify the name of the variable that defines the time and the variable that defines the event with the code to be used for the occurrence of the event, as follows:

```
stset time,fa(death=1)
```

Output

```
      failure event:  death == 1
obs. time interval:  (0, time]
 exit on or before:  failure
```

```
-------------------------------------------------------------------------------
     87   total observations
      5   observations end on or before enter()
-------------------------------------------------------------------------------
     82   observations remaining, representing
     43   failures in single-record/single-failure data
   2385   total analysis time at risk and under observation
                                        at risk from t =        0
                           earliest observed entry t =          0
                               last observed exit t =          99
```

We defined the time-of-survival variable at the beginning; in this case it was defined with the name *time*. After the comma, the occurrence of the event of interest is indicated with the command **fa** followed by a parenthesis to indicate the variable for the event of interest and the code that indicates when the event occurs.

An estimation of survival probability is obtained in Stata with the *ltable* command, as is demonstrated in the following:

ltable time

Output

Interval		Beg. Total	Deaths	Lost	Survival	Std. Error	[95% Conf. Int.]	
0	1	87	5	0	0.9425	0.0250	0.8674	0.9757
1	2	82	8	0	0.8506	0.0382	0.7566	0.9104
2	3	74	5	0	0.7931	0.0434	0.6919	0.8642
3	4	69	2	0	0.7701	0.0451	0.6667	0.8451
4	5	67	1	0	0.7586	0.0459	0.6542	0.8354
5	6	66	5	0	0.7011	0.0491	0.5930	0.7856
6	7	61	4	0	0.6552	0.0510	0.5453	0.7446
7	8	57	2	0	0.6322	0.0517	0.5218	0.7238
8	9	55	3	0	0.5977	0.0526	0.4870	0.6920
9	10	52	1	0	0.5862	0.0528	0.4755	0.6813
10	11	51	2	0	0.5632	0.0532	0.4527	0.6597
12	13	49	1	0	0.5517	0.0533	0.4414	0.6489
13	14	48	1	0	0.5402	0.0534	0.4302	0.6380
17	18	47	1	0	0.5287	0.0535	0.4190	0.6270
20	21	46	2	0	0.5057	0.0536	0.3967	0.6049
21	22	44	1	0	0.4943	0.0536	0.3857	0.5938
22	23	43	1	0	0.4828	0.0536	0.3747	0.5826
23	24	42	1	0	0.4713	0.0535	0.3637	0.5714
25	26	41	1	0	0.4598	0.0534	0.3529	0.5601
27	28	40	1	0	0.4483	0.0533	0.3420	0.5488
28	29	39	2	0	0.4253	0.0530	0.3205	0.5260
34	35	37	2	0	0.4023	0.0526	0.2993	0.5029
35	36	35	2	0	0.3793	0.0520	0.2783	0.4797
37	38	33	1	0	0.3678	0.0517	0.2678	0.4680

38	39	32	1	0	0.3563	0.0513	0.2575	0.4562
39	40	31	5	0	0.2989	0.0491	0.2067	0.3964
40	41	26	1	0	0.2874	0.0485	0.1967	0.3843
41	42	25	1	0	0.2759	0.0479	0.1868	0.3721
43	44	24	1	0	0.2644	0.0473	0.1770	0.3598
44	45	23	2	0	0.2414	0.0459	0.1577	0.3350
45	46	21	1	0	0.2299	0.0451	0.1481	0.3225
46	47	20	1	0	0.2184	0.0443	0.1387	0.3099
47	48	19	1	0	0.2069	0.0434	0.1293	0.2972
48	49	18	1	0	0.1954	0.0425	0.1200	0.2844
49	50	17	1	0	0.1839	0.0415	0.1109	0.2715
50	51	16	1	0	0.1724	0.0405	0.1019	0.2585
52	53	15	1	0	0.1609	0.0394	0.0930	0.2454
53	54	14	1	0	0.1494	0.0382	0.0842	0.2322
55	56	13	1	0	0.1379	0.0370	0.0756	0.2188
59	60	12	1	0	0.1264	0.0356	0.0671	0.2053
60	61	11	1	0	0.1149	0.0342	0.0589	0.1916
61	62	10	1	0	0.1034	0.0327	0.0508	0.1778
70	71	9	1	0	0.0920	0.0310	0.0430	0.1637
71	72	8	1	0	0.0805	0.0292	0.0354	0.1494
73	74	7	1	0	0.0690	0.0272	0.0282	0.1349
78	79	6	1	0	0.0575	0.0250	0.0213	0.1200
81	82	5	1	0	0.0460	0.0225	0.0150	0.1047
84	85	4	1	0	0.0345	0.0196	0.0092	0.0889
89	90	3	1	0	0.0230	0.0161	0.0044	0.0725
95	96	2	1	0	0.0115	0.0114	0.0010	0.0558
99	100	1	1	0	0.0000	.	.	.

Note: The command *ltable* is followed by the variable that indicates the observation time.

After running the *stset* command, the *sts graph* command can be used in Stata to construct the $S(t)$ graph using the KM method, as illustrated in Figure 10.3.

10.6 Hazard Function

Another way to assess the time of occurrence of an event is by using the *hazard function*, which is denoted by $h(t)$. This function is defined as the instantaneous risk of occurrence of the event of interest after a time, t, given that this event did not occur during at least a single time t. To estimate the hazard function using the KM method, in a given time interval $(t_{(j)}, t_{(j+1)})$, a similar process is used to compute the incidence density:

$$\hat{h}(t) = \frac{f_j}{r_j * \tau_j} = \frac{\text{cases}}{\text{person-time}}$$

where τ_j indicates the size of the interval $(t_{(j)}, t_{(j+1)})$, that is, $\tau_j = t_{(j+1)} - t_{(j)}$. According to the time unit that is used, the product $r_j * \tau_j$ indicates person-time (i.e., person-years,

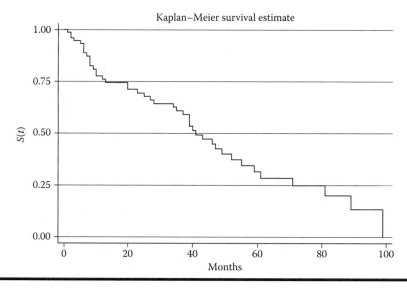

Figure 10.3   Survival function using the Kaplan–Meier method.

person-weeks, person-days, etc.). The estimation of the hazard probabilities can also be obtained with the *ltable* command, but we add the *hazard* option. For example, using the previous data, the command is as follows:

```
ltable time, hazard
```

Output

Interval		Beg. Total	Cum. Failure	Std. Error	Hazard	Std. Error	[95% Conf. Int.]	
0	1	87	0.0575	0.0250	0.0592	0.0265	0.0073	0.1110
1	2	82	0.1494	0.0382	0.1026	0.0362	0.0316	0.1735
2	3	74	0.2069	0.0434	0.0699	0.0313	0.0087	0.1312
3	4	69	0.2299	0.0451	0.0294	0.0208	0.0000	0.0702
4	5	67	0.2414	0.0459	0.0150	0.0150	0.0000	0.0445
5	6	66	0.2989	0.0491	0.0787	0.0352	0.0098	0.1477
6	7	61	0.3448	0.0510	0.0678	0.0339	0.0014	0.1342
7	8	57	0.3678	0.0517	0.0357	0.0252	0.0000	0.0852
8	9	55	0.4023	0.0526	0.0561	0.0324	0.0000	0.1195
9	10	52	0.4138	0.0528	0.0194	0.0194	0.0000	0.0575
10	11	51	0.4368	0.0532	0.0400	0.0283	0.0000	0.0954
12	13	49	0.4483	0.0533	0.0206	0.0206	0.0000	0.0610
13	14	48	0.4598	0.0534	0.0211	0.0211	0.0000	0.0623
17	18	47	0.4713	0.0535	0.0215	0.0215	0.0000	0.0637
20	21	46	0.4943	0.0536	0.0444	0.0314	0.0000	0.1060
21	22	44	0.5057	0.0536	0.0230	0.0230	0.0000	0.0680
22	23	43	0.5172	0.0536	0.0235	0.0235	0.0000	0.0696

23	24	42	0.5287	0.0535	0.0241	0.0241	0.0000	0.0713
25	26	41	0.5402	0.0534	0.0247	0.0247	0.0000	0.0731
27	28	40	0.5517	0.0533	0.0253	0.0253	0.0000	0.0749
28	29	39	0.5747	0.0530	0.0526	0.0372	0.0000	0.1255
34	35	37	0.5977	0.0526	0.0556	0.0393	0.0000	0.1325
35	36	35	0.6207	0.0520	0.0588	0.0416	0.0000	0.1403
37	38	33	0.6322	0.0517	0.0308	0.0308	0.0000	0.0911
38	39	32	0.6437	0.0513	0.0317	0.0317	0.0000	0.0940
39	40	31	0.7011	0.0491	0.1754	0.0782	0.0223	0.3286
40	41	26	0.7126	0.0485	0.0392	0.0392	0.0000	0.1161
41	42	25	0.7241	0.0479	0.0408	0.0408	0.0000	0.1208
43	44	24	0.7356	0.0473	0.0426	0.0425	0.0000	0.1259
44	45	23	0.7586	0.0459	0.0909	0.0642	0.0000	0.2168
45	46	21	0.7701	0.0451	0.0488	0.0488	0.0000	0.1444
46	47	20	0.7816	0.0443	0.0513	0.0513	0.0000	0.1518
47	48	19	0.7931	0.0434	0.0541	0.0540	0.0000	0.1600
48	49	18	0.8046	0.0425	0.0571	0.0571	0.0000	0.1691
49	50	17	0.8161	0.0415	0.0606	0.0606	0.0000	0.1793
50	51	16	0.8276	0.0405	0.0645	0.0645	0.0000	0.1909
52	53	15	0.8391	0.0394	0.0690	0.0689	0.0000	0.2041
53	54	14	0.8506	0.0382	0.0741	0.0740	0.0000	0.2192
55	56	13	0.8621	0.0370	0.0800	0.0799	0.0000	0.2367
59	60	12	0.8736	0.0356	0.0870	0.0869	0.0000	0.2572
60	61	11	0.8851	0.0342	0.0952	0.0951	0.0000	0.2817
61	62	10	0.8966	0.0327	0.1053	0.1051	0.0000	0.3113
70	71	9	0.9080	0.0310	0.1176	0.1174	0.0000	0.3478
71	72	8	0.9195	0.0292	0.1333	0.1330	0.0000	0.3941
73	74	7	0.9310	0.0272	0.1538	0.1534	0.0000	0.4545
78	79	6	0.9425	0.0250	0.1818	0.1811	0.0000	0.5367
81	82	5	0.9540	0.0225	0.2222	0.2208	0.0000	0.6551
84	85	4	0.9655	0.0196	0.2857	0.2828	0.0000	0.8400
89	90	3	0.9770	0.0161	0.4000	0.3919	0.0000	1.1681
95	96	2	0.9885	0.0114	0.6667	0.6285	0.0000	1.8986
99	100	1	1.0000	.	2.0000	0.0000	2.0000	2.0000

To graphically represent $h(t)$ through the KM method, the same command for $S(t)$ is used, but we add the hazard option (**sts graph, hazard**). The output of this command is illustrated in Figure 10.4.

10.7 Relationship between $S(t)$ and $h(t)$

Assuming that the time of observation, T, is a random variable in the survival analysis setting, then, as a consequence, the following functions exist:

$f(t)$: the probability density function of T
$F(t)$: the probability cumulative function of $f(t)$

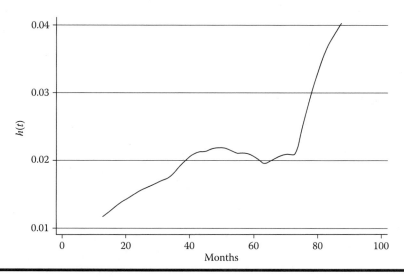

Figure 10.4   Hazard function.

It has been shown that there is a mathematical relationship between these survival and hazard functions, the specifics of which are as follows (Collett, 2003):

a. $f(t) = \dfrac{\partial F(t)}{\partial t} = \dfrac{\partial \left(1 - S(t)\right)}{\partial t} = -S'(t)$

b. $h(t) = \lim_{\Delta t \to 0} \dfrac{\Pr\left(t + \Delta t > T > t \mid T > t\right)}{\Delta t} = \dfrac{f(t)}{S(t)}$

c. $H(t) = \displaystyle\int_{0}^{t} h(u)\,\partial u = \int_{0}^{t} \dfrac{f(u)}{S(u)}\,\partial u = -\int_{0}^{t} \dfrac{1}{S(u)}\left(\dfrac{\partial S(u)}{\partial u}\right)\partial u = -\ln\left(S(t)\right)$

where $S'(t)$ indicates the derivative of $S(t)$ and $H(t)$, the cumulative hazard function.

10.8 Cumulative Hazard Function

The following methods are available for determining the cumulative hazard function:

1. The KM method:

$$\widehat{H}(t) = -\text{Ln}\left(\hat{S}(t)\right) = -\text{Ln}\left(\prod_{t(i) \le t}\left(\dfrac{r_i - f_i}{r_i}\right)\right) = \sum_{t(i) \le t} -\text{Ln}\left(1 - \dfrac{f_i}{r_i}\right)$$

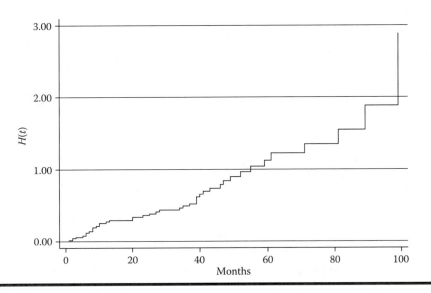

Figure 10.5 Nelson–Aelen cumulative hazard estimate.

2. The Nelson–Aalen method:

$$\widetilde{H}(t) = \sum_{t(i) \leq t} \frac{f_i}{r_i}$$

The estimate of $H(t)$ using the Nelson–Aelen method will always be greater than or equal to that which is generated using the KM method. When the number of subjects at risk at any given time is large, the two estimates are basically equal. Based on the Nelson–Aalen method, we can obtain the survival function with the following expression:

$$S(\widetilde{t}) = e^{(-H(t))}$$

The graphic representation of the cumulative hazard [$H(t)$] using the Nelson–Aalen method is programmed in Stata using the following command to create Figure 10.5:

```
sts graph, cumhaz
```

10.9 Median Survival Time and Percentiles

The minimum survival time in which the probabilities are less than 50% is identified by the median survival time {$t(50) = \min(\text{time}|S(t) < 50\%)$}. In Stata this time is obtained as follows:

```
stci, median
```

Output

```
    failure _d:  death == 1
  analysis time _t:  time

          |  no. of
          |  subjects    50%    Std. Err.     [95% Conf. Interval]
----------+--------------------------------------------------------------
  total   |    82        41     3.705979                   34          55
```

Note: The **median** option is added.

If an estimate of other times, based on percentiles $[(1-S(t)]$, is required, we use the option **p** with the integer that indicates the percentile. For example, for the percentiles 25 and 75, the Stata commands are as follows:

```
stci, p(25)
```

Output

```
          |  no. of
          |  subjects    25%    Std. Err.    [95% Conf. Interval]
----------+-------------------------------------------------------------

  total   |    82        13     6.687969                  8          28
```

```
stci, p(75)
```

Output

```
          |  no. of
          |  subjects    75%    Std. Err.    [95% Conf.  Interval]
----------+--------------------------------------------------------------
  total   |    82        71     12.37697                  52          .
```

Note: In the previous case, the 25th percentile indicates the minimum time for which the survival probabilities are less than 75%. The 75th percentile indicates the minimum time for which the survival probabilities are less than 25%.

10.10 Comparison of Survival Curves

To compare the overall experience of two or more survival curves, you can use different tests of significance. Initially, it is recommended that a graph of $S_i(t)$ by different subgroups of the stratum be constructed. The Stata programming for visualizing different survival curves in the same plot, using the KM method, uses the option *by* after the *sts graph* command. For example, using the previous database, the survival curves by sex are graphically obtained with the following command to create Figure 10.6:

```
sts graph, by(sex)
```

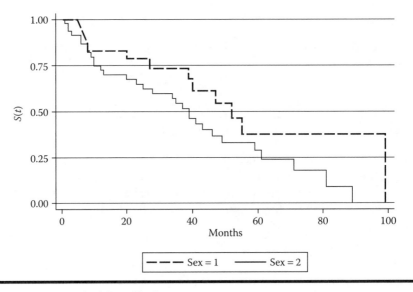

Figure 10.6   Survival function by sex.

To obtain the median survival time in different subgroups, the option *by* can also be used after the *stci* command. For example, the command line for finding the median time by sex would be

```
stci, median by(sex)
```

Output

sex	no. of subjects	50%	Std. Err.	[95% Conf.	Interval]
1	31	52	5.187957	27	.
2	51	39	3.999146	23	49
total	82	41	3.705979	34	55

10.11 Proportional Hazards Assumption

The application of certain significance tests to evaluate hazard functions depends on the behavior of these functions among the study groups over time. If the ratio of hazard functions is constant over time $h_1(t)/h_2(t)$ = constant, it is said that the hazards are proportional (proportional hazards). For example, using the previous database, the hazard function curves by sex are graphically obtained with the following command to create Figure 10.7:

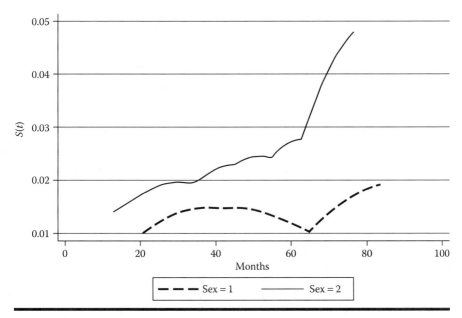

Figure 10.7 Hazard function by sex.

```
sts graph, by(sex) hazard
```

A *proportional hazards (PH)* assessment can be performed through the pattern observed in the survival function curves. It is a necessary but not sufficient condition that the curves not cross over time, suggesting that the PH assumption is met. An alternate way to evaluate this assumption graphically is to determine whether the function $\ln\{-\ln[S(t)]\}$ is kept parallel through time. For example, for programming this function we use the following command to create Figure 10.8:

```
stphplot, by(sex)
```

10.12 Significance Assessment

Hypothesis testing can be performed to compare the survival curves of different groups. There are several methods that can be used to evaluate these curves, which include the log-rank test, the Wilcoxon–Gehan–Breslow (WGB) test, and the Tarone–Ware test. A log-rank test is recommended when the condition of PH is fulfilled, while a Wilcoxon test is recommended when the condition of PH is not fulfilled.

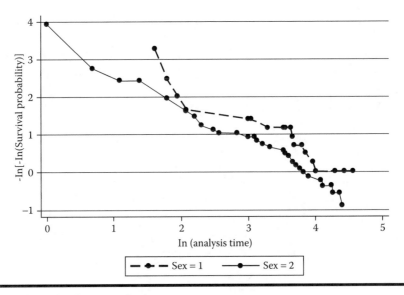

Figure 10.8 **ln{−ln(S(t))} plot by sex.**

10.12.1 Log-Rank Test

To compare the survival curves, the log-rank test assumes the following null hypothesis:

$$H_0 : S_1(t) = S_2(t)$$

To evaluate the survival curves with the log-rank test, the following contingency table is constructed at each time $t_{(j)}$:

Group	Events	No Events	Number at Risk
1	f_{1j}	$r_{1j} - f_{1j}$	r_{1j}
2	f_{2j}	$r_{2j} - f_{2j}$	r_{2j}
Total	f_j	$r_j - f_j$	r_{1j}

Under the null hypothesis of no association between the type of group and the occurrence of the event, you can determine the expected events in each group and compare with the observed event with the following statistics:

$$\frac{U^2_L}{V_L} \sim \chi^2_{(1)}$$

where:

$U_L = \Sigma w_i (f_{1j} - e_{1j})$ defines the weighted difference (observed events minus expected events $E(f_{1j}) = e_{1j}$, under H_0) with equal weights ($w_i = 1$) over time

$V_L = \Sigma v_{ij}$ determines the sum of the variances under the hypergeometric distribution $v_{ij} = \mathrm{Var}(f_{1j}) = r_{1j} {}^* r_{\mathrm{II}j} {}^* f_j {}^* (r_j - f_j)/r^2{}_j {}^* (r_j - 1)$

The Stata command for a log-rank test is:

```
sts test sex, logrank
```

Output

```
Log-rank test for equality of survivor functions
          |    Events          Events
sex       |   observed        expected
----------+-----------------------------
1         |      12             17.84
2         |      31             25.16
----------+-----------------------------
Total     |      43             43.00
                         chi2(1)  =      3.48
                         Pr>chi2  =     0.0620
```

According to the log-rank test performed, there is evidence in favor of H_0: $S_1(t) = S_2(t)$ (P-value = .062). However, some users might even consider this statistical evidence as marginally significant ($0.05 \leq P\text{-value} < .1$).

10.12.2 Wilcoxon–Gehan–Breslow Test

The Wilcoxon–Gehan–Breslow (WGB) test is also based on the null hypothesis

$$H_0 : S_1(t) = S_2(t)$$

To perform this test, the following statistic is computed:

$$\frac{U^2_{\mathrm{WGB}}}{V_{\mathrm{WGB}}} \sim \chi^2_{(1)}$$

where:

$$U_{\mathrm{WGB}} = \sum w_j * (f_{1j} - e_{1j}); \quad w_j = r_j$$

$$V_{\mathrm{WGW}} = \sum w_j^2 * v_{1j}$$

The difference between the U_W statistic and the statistics of the log-rank test is that $(f_{ij} - e_{ij})$ is being weighted by r_j. As time increases, the r_j decreases; therefore, individuals with very high values in the observation times will have less weight. The Stata command for this test is

```
sts test sex, wilcoxon
```

Output

```
Wilcoxon (Breslow) test for equality of survivor functions
```

sex	Events observed	Events expected	Sum of ranks
1	12	17.84	-208
2	31	25.16	208
Total	43	43.00	0

```
            chi2(1) =    2.23
            Pr>chi2 =  0.1350
```

According to the Wilcoxon test, there is evidence in favor of the statement H_0: $S_1(t) = S_2(t)$ (*P*-value > .1).

10.12.3 Tarone–Ware Test

The Tarone–Ware test is similar to the WGB test, but the weighting factor is r_j^2. The Stata command for this is as follows:

```
sts test sex, tware
```

Output

```
Tarone-Ware test for equality of survivor functions
```

sex	Events observed	Events expected	Sum of ranks
1	12	17.84	-31.88649
2	31	25.16	31.88649
Total	43	43.00	0

```
            chi2(1) =    2.63
            Pr>chi2 =  0.1049
```

According to the Tarone–Ware test, there is evidence in favor of the statement H_0: $S_1(t) = S_2(t)$ (*P*-value > .10).

10.13 Cox Proportional Hazards Model

To evaluate the effect of an exposure on the hazard function, controlling for the presence of potential confounding variables, we can use the *Cox proportional hazards model* (Royston and Lambert, 2011), as follows:

$$h(t, X) = h_0(t) * e^{\beta_E * E + \sum \beta_i X_i}$$

where:

E defines the exposure variable of interest

X_i defines the group of independent or predictor variables (it includes potential confounding variables and interaction terms)

β_i defines the group of coefficients of the predictor variables

$h_0(t)$ defines the immediate risk in time t. This function depends on the time and indicates the risk at initial conditions ($E = 0$, $X_i = 0$) or in average conditions when the predictor variables are centralized ($E = 0$, $X_i - \overline{X}$)

The predictor variables can be time dependent (e.g., age, blood pressure), but in this book, we are analyzing only those variables that are not time dependent. One of the most important uses of this model in epidemiologic studies is to estimate the hazard ratio (HR) adjusted for potential confounding variables. For example, assuming that the hazard between two persons having different exposure levels is obtained by the Cox model without interaction terms, the HR is estimated as follows:

First person ($E = 1$):

$$h_1(t; x) = h_0(t) * e^{(\beta_E + \beta_1 X_1 + \cdots + \beta_k X_k)}$$

Second person ($E = 0$):

$$h_2(t; x') = h_0(t) * e^{(\beta_1 X_1' + \dots + \beta_K X_K')}$$

as a consequence,

$$\text{HR} = \frac{h_1(t; x)}{h_2(t; x')}$$

$$\text{HR} = e^{\left[\beta_E + \beta_1 * (X_1 - X_1') + \beta_2 * (X_2 - X_2') + \cdots + \beta_k (X_k - X_k')\right]}$$

If we assume that the difference between both persons is only the exposure, then:

$$(X_1 = X_1'),\ (X_2 = X_2'),\dots,(X_k = X_k')$$

As a consequence, the adjusted HR is obtained with the following:

$$HR_{adjusted} = e^{\beta_E}$$

During the HR estimation, the $h_0(t)$ function is canceled. We assume that the HR remains constant over time; therefore, the HR varies only according to the value of the predictor variables. This process of obtaining the adjusted HR is similar to that used in evaluating the adjusted OR and RR of the logistic and Poisson regression models, respectively.

The Stata commands to evaluate the interaction terms in the Cox regression model is as follows:

```
. quietly xi: stcox i.sex*i.stage
. estimates store model1
. quietly xi: stcox i.sex i.stage
. lrtest model1 .
```

Output

```
Likelihood-ratio test              LR chi2(2)   =      1.62
(Assumption: . nested in model1)   Prob > chi2 =      0.4440
```

The results show that there is no evidence of any significant interaction terms in the Cox model (P-value $> .10$). Now, to assess the effect of potential confounding variables, we need to compare the crude and adjusted HRs. To estimate the crude HR, *stcox* is used, as can be seen in the following:

```
stcox b1.sex
```

Output

```
------------------------------------------------------------------------
   _t | Haz. Ratio Std. Err.    z    P>|z|   [95% Conf. Interval]
-------+----------------------------------------------------------------
 2.sex | 1.906899   0.6747282 1.82  0.068   0.9531086   3.815161
------------------------------------------------------------------------
```

Note: The use of $b1$ before the predictor is to indicate that the category with a code equal to 1 is the reference category.

The HR between sexes adjusted for stage is estimated with the following Stata command:

```
stcox b1.sex b1.stage
```

Output

```
-----------------------------------------------------------------
      _t | Haz. Ratio   Std. Err.    z    P>|z|   [95% Conf. Interval]
---------+-------------------------------------------------------
   2.sex |   1.894716   0.690035   1.75   0.079   0.9279952    3.868499
         |
   stage |
       2 |   1.472089   0.5575111  1.02   0.307   0.7007552    3.092446
       3 |   3.766573   1.596584   3.13   0.002   1.641108     8.644817
-----------------------------------------------------------------
```

This example indicates that tumor stage is not a confounding variable in the association of *sex* and cancer mortality because the difference between the estimated HR_{Crude} (1.91) and the estimated $HR_{Adjusted}$ (1.89) is very small.

10.14 Assessment of the Proportional Hazards Assumption

If the condition of PH is fulfilled, there should not be an interaction between *time* and the exposure variable (E). To confirm this pattern, you can use the Cox model, as is demonstrated by the following:

$$h(t; x_1) = h_0(t) * e^{\beta_E * E + \beta_X * X}$$

where:

$$X = E * \ln(\text{time})$$

If the PH condition is met, then $\beta_E = 0$. Therefore, the expectation is that the interaction variable X would not be statistically significant to provide evidence that the PH assumption is met.

There are several methods for assessing the PH assumption, which are based on the quantities known as residuals. A description of these methods can be read in Collett (2003). Stata uses Schoenfeld residuals, or partial residuals, as its method for assessing PH. This method can be used with the option *phtest* after running *stcox*, as is demonstrated in the following:

```
quietly: stcox i.sex i.stage
estat phtest, detail
```

Output

```
Test of proportional-hazards assumption
```

```
Time:   Time
---------------------------------------------------------------------
              |      rho        chi2         df        Prob>chi2
--------------+------------------------------------------------------
1b.sex        |       .           .           1            .
2.sex         |    0.10298      0.46          1          0.4954
1b.stage      |       .           .           1            .
2.stage       |   -0.03693      0.06          1          0.8142
3.stage       |   -0.09269      0.33          1          0.5671
--------------+------------------------------------------------------
global test   |                 0.80          3          0.8483
---------------------------------------------------------------------
```

The data suggest that the condition of PH is fulfilled for both predictors simultaneously (P-value > .10).

10.15 Survival Function Estimation Using the Cox Proportional Hazards Model

Using the Cox model, we can obtain the survival function as follows:

$$S(t,E,x,\beta) = e^{-H(E,t,x,\beta)} = e^{-g(E,x,\beta)H_0(t)} = \left[e^{-H_0(t)}\right]^{g(E,x,\beta)} = \left[S_0(t)\right]^{g(x,\beta)}$$

where:

$$g(E,x,\beta) = e^{\beta_E * E + \sum \beta_i X_i}$$

$$S_0(t) = e^{-H_0(t)}$$

Therefore, for visualizing the survival curves by sex at stage 3 (stage = 3) after running the Cox model, the following sequences of commands is used to create Figure 10.9:

```
quietly xi: stcox b1.sex b1.stage
stcurve , survival at1(sex=1 stage=3) at2(sex=2 stage=3)
```

10.16 Stratified Cox Proportional Hazards Model

If the predictors do not satisfy the PH assumption, we recommend using the stratified Cox model, which is expressed as follows:

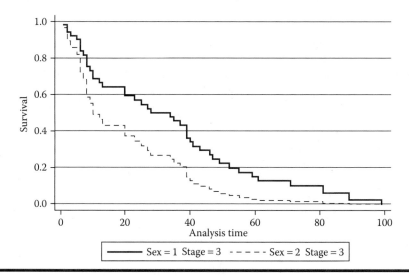

Figure 10.9 Survival curves by sex at stage 3.

$$h_g(t, X) = h_{0g}(t) e^{\beta_E * E + \sum \beta_i * X_i}$$

where *g* indicates the stratum.

It is necessary to first identify all the predictors that do not satisfy the PH. With these predictor categories, strata are formed. For example, if the *stage* variable does not satisfy the PH assumption, the Cox model can be stratified by *stage* levels. In Stata the command line for the stratified Cox model using the previous data would have the variable *sex* as the sole predictor, as follows:

```
xi: stcox  b1.sex, strata(stage) nolog
```

Output

```
Stratified Cox regr.  -- Breslow method for ties
No. of subjects =            82         Number of obs  =           82
No. of failures =            43
Time at risk    =          2385
                                        LR chi2(1)     =         2.84
Log likelihood  =   -98.460443          Prob > chi2    =       0.0919
-----------------------------------------------------------------------
    _t | Haz. Ratio  Std. Err.    z   P>|z|  [95% Conf. Interval]
-------+---------------------------------------------------------------
 2.sex |   1.818963  0.6677337 1.63 0.103   0.8858321   3.73505
-----------------------------------------------------------------------
                                             Stratified by stage
```

A slight variation is observed between the HR stratified by stage ($HR_{stratified\ by\ stage}$: 1.82, 95% CI: 0.89, 3.74) and the adjusted HR ($HR_{adjusted\ by\ stage}$: 1.89, 95% CI = 0.93, 3.87).

There are other applications of survival analysis that can be explored in Stata, including time-dependent predictors, competing risks regression, parametric survival models, and multilevel parametric regression. These topics are beyond the scope of this book, but an extensive review of survival analysis can be found in Collett (2003), Peace (2009), Royston and Lambert (2011), and Wienke (2011).

Chapter 11

Analysis of Correlated Data

Aim: Upon completing the chapter, the learner should be able to fit a linear regression with correlated data.

11.1 Regression Models with Correlated Data

When the measurements are part of a group of individuals, then it is possible that these measurements will be correlated. For example, patients receiving medical care in a hospital (private or public) and who are assigned to a doctor (generalist or specialist), it is possible that the treatments that these patients receive will be very similar. The patients are observed nested within certain type of doctors and hospitals.

Another example of correlated data is in cross-sectional studies, when a complex sampling design of households is used (Figure 11.1); the possibility exists that the responses of the people who reside on the same census block about lifestyle habits will be similar.

Another situation in which there might be correlated data is when repeated measurements are made; for example, the different weights of a single child at different visits to his or her pediatrician. There are various alternatives for analyzing these data, and which alternatives to use will depend on the objectives of the investigator. One alternative is to analyze the independent measurements separately, which results in a loss of information and statistical power. For example, assume the following data with regard to 20 different children, each one visiting his or her pediatrician three different times, being weighed at each visit, and information on whether they practice a sport on a regular basis (1 = yes vs. 0 = no):

	id	weight1	weight2	weight3	sport
1.	1	66	67	68	0
2.	2	71	71	65	0
3.	3	70	66	62	0
4.	4	64	62	66	1
5.	5	67	66	68	1
6.	6	65	64	65	1
7.	7	67	67	63	0
8.	8	65	66	66	1
9.	9	69	70	68	0
10.	10	63	62	63	1
11.	11	61	60	60	1
12.	12	66	68	68	1
13.	13	68	68	70	0
14.	14	67	69	65	0
15.	15	65	67	63	1
16.	16	64	62	64	1
17.	17	65	64	55	0
18.	18	65	65	66	0
19.	19	64	63	62	1
20.	20	67	66	63	0

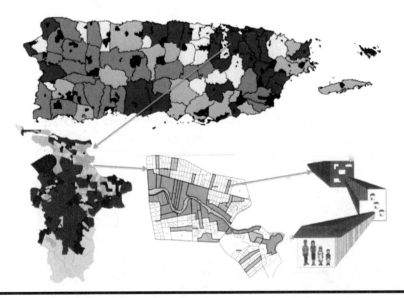

Figure 11.1 Sampling design in Puerto Rico.

To perform the analysis with independent measurements, assuming that the objective is to compare the average weight by type of sport, we could carry out a simple linear regression analysis of the weight of each child, using the following command lines at each visit:

For the first visit:

```
reg weight1 sport
```

Output

```
    Source |       SS       df       MS              Number of obs   =        20
-----------+------------------------------           F(1, 18)        =     14.20
     Model |     48.05        1        48.05          Prob > F        =    0.0014
  Residual |      60.9       18   3.38333333          R-squared       =    0.4410
-----------+------------------------------           Adj R-squared   =    0.4100
     Total |    108.95       19   5.73421053          Root MSE        =    1.8394


------------------------------------------------------------------------------
   weight1 |      Coef.   Std. Err.      t    P>|t|     [95% Conf. Interval]
-----------+------------------------------------------------------------------
     sport |      -3.1    .8225975    -3.77   0.001    -4.828213    -1.371787
     _cons |      67.5    .5816643   116.05   0.000     66.27797     68.72203
------------------------------------------------------------------------------
```

The results show a significant effect of the predictor sport on mean weight at visit 1 (*P*-value = .001). The estimated regression coefficient for the predictor *sport* is the difference between the mean weights by sport in visit 1. The following command line can be used to compute the observed mean weight by sport:

```
table sport, c(mean weight1)
```

Output

```
-----------------------
    sport | mean(weight1)
----------+------------
        0 |          67.5
        1 |          64.4
-----------------------
```

The difference in the mean weights at visit 1 is −3.1, so the children who practice regularly a sport weigh less, on average, than those who do not practice regularly a sport. To explore the differences in mean weight in each visit, a line can be drawn between the estimated weights from a linear regression model by sport. For example, in the first visit the following Stata commands for visualizing this line can be used to create Figure 11.2:

```
predict weight1exp
twoway (line weight1exp sport, sort), ytitle(Mean weight)
xtitle(Sport) xlabel(0(1)1) legend(off)
```

We repeat the previous steps for the second visit:

```
reg weight2 sport
```

Output

```
    Source |      SS       df       MS         Number of obs  =       20
-----------+-----------------------------       F(1, 18)       =     9.24
     Model |    54.45       1      54.45        Prob > F       =   0.0071
  Residual |    106.1      18 5.89444444        R-squared      =   0.3391
-----------+-----------------------------       Adj R-squared  =   0.3024
     Total |   160.55      19       8.45        Root MSE       =   2.4278


----------------------------------------------------------------------------

   weight2 |Coef.   Std. Err.    t      P>|t|    [95% Conf. Interval]
-----------+----------------------------------------------------------------
     sport |-3.3    1.085766   -3.04   0.007    -5.581111   -1.018889
     _cons |67.3     .7677529   87.66   0.000    65.68701    68.91299
----------------------------------------------------------------------------
```

```
table sport, c(mean weight2)
```

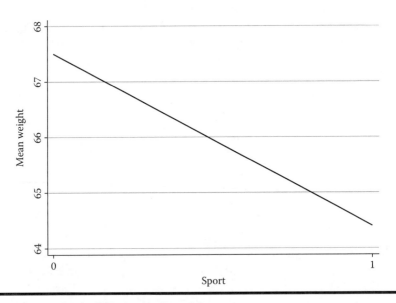

Figure 11.2   Mean weight in the first visit.

Output

```
-----------------------------
  sport |  mean(weight2)
--------+--------------------
      0 |             67.3
      1 |               64
-----------------------------
```

The results also show a significant effect of the predictor sport on mean weight at visit 2 (*P*-value = .007). The difference in the mean weights at the second visit is −3.3; children who practice regularly a sport weight less, on average, than those who do not practice regularly a sport. To draw the estimated weight by sport at visit 2, the following Stata commands are used to create Figure 11.3:

```
predict weight2exp
twoway (line weight2exp sport, sort), ytitle(Mean weight)
xtitle(Sport) xlabel(0(1)1) legend(off)
```

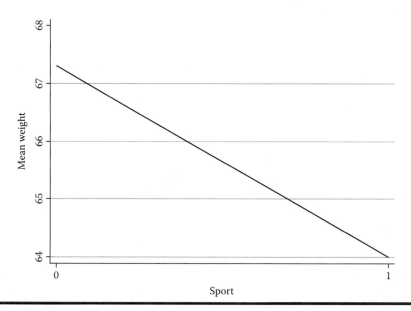

Figure 11.3   Mean weight in the second visit.

The Stata commands on the third visit are:

```
reg weight3 sport
```

Output

```
      Source |    SS     df       MS              Number of obs  =        20
-------------+----------------------------        F(1, 18)       =      0.00
       Model |     0      1        0              Prob > F       =    1.0000
    Residual |   219     18   12.1666667          R-squared      =    0.0000
-------------+----------------------------        Adj R-squared  =   -0.0556
       Total |   219     19   11.5263158          Root MSE       =    3.4881


-----------------------------------------------------------------------------
     weight3 |  Coef.  Std. Err.     t    P>|t|   [95% Conf. Interval]
-------------+---------------------------------------------------------------
       sport |      0  1.559915    0.00   1.000   -3.277259    3.277259
       _cons |   64.5  1.103026   58.48   0.000    62.18263    66.81737
-----------------------------------------------------------------------------
```

```
table sport, c(mean weight3)
```

Output

```
-------------------------
    sport |  mean(weight3)
----------+--------------
        0 |          64.5
        1 |          64.5
-------------------------
```

The results do not show a significant effect of the predictor sport on mean weight at visit 3 (*P*-value > .1). There is no difference in the mean weights at the third visit. To draw the estimated weight by sport on the third visit, the following Stata commands are used to create Figure 11.4:

```
predict weight3exp
twoway (line weight3exp sex, sort), ytitle(Mean weight)
xtitle(Sport) xlabel(0(1)1) legend(off)
```

11.2 Mixed Models

The other alternative for analyzing correlated data is to use mixed models or multi-level models that allow us to correct the statistical relationship due to the potential correlation between measurements. For example, the simplest scheme of correlation is the repeated measures study; the same subject is measured several times, as illustrated in Figure 11.5.

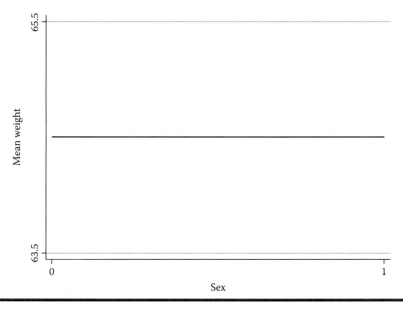

Figure 11.4   Mean weight in the third visit.

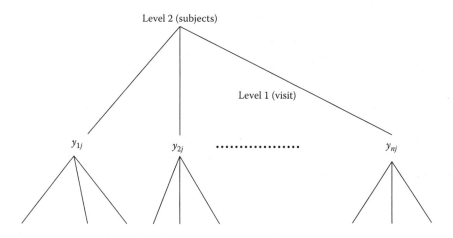

y_{ij} indicates the value of Y in the *j*th visit for the *i*th subject.

Level 1 refers to the set of weights of each subject on different visits.

Level 2 refers to the set of subjects.

Figure 11.5   Repeated measures of weight in the same subject.

Mixed models can be expressed in various forms to explain the expected value of the *main outcome* (*Y*) of the study. The construction of these models depends on the following variations:

1. $\bar{Y}_i$ may be different between subjects at baseline (variability between measurements).
2. $\bar{Y}_i$ may change according to the conditions in each subject (variability within measurements).

When an association is established between a continuous random variable, *Y*, and a quantitative variable, *X*, through a simple linear regression model, $\mu_{Y|X} = \beta_0 + \beta_1 * X$, in a mixed model approach, the intercept (β_0) and the slope (β_1) could be fixed or random. The following table indicates the possible combinations of these alternatives:

Intercept (β_0)	Slope (β_1)
Fixed	Fixed
Fixed	Random
Random	Fixed
Random	Random

Based on the previous example of the estimated weights by sport, we need to identify the possible patterns of the linear relationships. According to the previous graphs, the respective patterns in the lines suggest a model with a random intercept considering the first two visits, similar slopes but different intercept; it means that the difference in the mean weight, between those who practice regularly a sport and those who do not, is independent of the visit. However, if the three visits are considered, a model with random intercept and slope is suggested; the difference in the mean weight, between those who practice sport and those who do not, is not independent of the visit.

11.3 Random Intercept

The definition of a linear mixed model with a random intercept is as follows (Rabe-Hesketh and Skrondal, 2005):

$$Y_{ij} = \beta_{0i} + \beta_1 * X_{ij} + e_{ij}$$

where:

$\beta_{0i} = \gamma_{00} + U_{0i}$ (random coefficient)

β_1 indicates the coefficients (fixed) associated to the predictor X

$U_{0i} \sim N\left(0, \sigma_{U_0}^2\right)$

γ_{00} indicates the average intercept in a design with two levels

σ_{u0}^2 indicates the variance of the intercept between subjects

The variance of Y_{ij} conditional on the value of X_{ij} is given by the following expression:

$$\mathrm{var}\left(Y_{ij}|X_{ij}\right) = \mathrm{var}\left(U_{0j}\right) + \mathrm{var}\left(\varepsilon_{ij}\right) = \sigma_{u0}^2 + \sigma_{\varepsilon}^2$$

where σ_{ε}^2 indicates the variance of Y within the subjects (variance of the residuals).

Using the data of the previous example, the correlation between two different visits $(j \neq j')$ of the ith subject is calculated through the covariance expression, as follows:

$$\mathrm{cov}\left(Y_{ij}, Y_{ij'}|X_{ij}, X_{ij'}\right) = \mathrm{var}\left(U_{0j}\right) = \sigma_{u0}^2$$

Therefore, the correlation between the measurements of Y in a subject, when Y is fitted by X, is defined with the following equation:

$$\rho\left(Y_{ij} \mid X_{ij}\right) = \frac{\mathrm{cov}\left(Y_{ij}, Y_{ij'} \mid X_{ij}, X_{ij'}\right)}{\mathrm{var}\left(Y_{ij} \mid X_{ij}\right)} = \frac{\sigma_{u0}^2}{\sigma_{u0}^2 + \sigma_{\varepsilon}^2}$$

This measurement is known as an intraclass correlation coefficient, which does not change according to the value of X.

11.4 Using the *mixed* and *gllamm* Commands with a Random Intercept

To run the mixed model with the assumption of a random intercept, we need the database to be in the long format. The following command needed to get a long database from a wide database is:

```
reshape long weight, i(id) j(visit)
```

After submitting this command, the database is changed as follows:

```
     +----------------------------------+
     | id    visit    weight    sport |
     |----------------------------------|
  1. | 1      1        66         0    |
  2. | 1      2        67         0    |
  3. | 1      3        68         0    |
  4. | 2      1        71         0    |
  5. | 2      2        71         0    |
     |----------------------------------|
  6. | 2      3        65         0    |
  7. | 3      1        70         0    |
  8. | 3      2        66         0    |
  9. | 3      3        62         0    |
 10. | 4      1        64         1    |
     |----------------------------------|
 11. | 4      2        62         1    |
 12. | 4      3        66         1    |
 13. | 5      1        67         1    |
 14. | 5      2        66         1    |
 15. | 5      3        68         1    |
     |----------------------------------|
 16. | 6      1        65         1    |
 17. | 6      2        64         1    |
 18. | 6      3        65         1    |
 19. | 7      1        67         0    |
 20. | 7      2        67         0    |
     |----------------------------------|
 21. | 7      3        63         0    |
 22. | 8      1        65         1    |
 23. | 8      2        66         1    |
 24. | 8      3        66         1    |
 25. | 9      1        69         0    |
     |----------------------------------|
 26. | 9      2        70         0    |
 27. | 9      3        68         0    |
 28. | 10     1        63         1    |
 29. | 10     2        62         1    |
 30. | 10     3        63         1    |
     |----------------------------------|
 31. | 11     1        61         1    |
 32. | 11     2        60         1    |
 33. | 11     3        60         1    |
 34. | 12     1        66         1    |
 35. | 12     2        68         1    |
     |----------------------------------|
```

```
36.  |  12        3        68        1  |
37.  |  13        1        68        0  |
38.  |  13        2        68        0  |
39.  |  13        3        70        0  |
40.  |  14        1        67        0  |
     |-----------------------------|
41.  |  14        2        69        0  |
42.  |  14        3        65        0  |
43.  |  15        1        65        1  |
44.  |  15        2        67        1  |
45.  |  15        3        63        1  |
     |-----------------------------|
46.  |  16        1        64        1  |
47.  |  16        2        62        1  |
48.  |  16        3        64        1  |
49.  |  17        1        65        0  |
50.  |  17        2        64        0  |
     |-----------------------------|
51.  |  17        3        55        0  |
52.  |  18        1        65        0  |
53.  |  18        2        65        0  |
54.  |  18        3        66        0  |
55.  |  19        1        64        1  |
     |-----------------------------|
56.  |  19        2        63        1  |
57.  |  19        3        62        1  |
58.  |  20        1        67        0  |
59.  |  20        2        66        0  |
60.  |  20        3        63        0  |
     +-----------------------------+
```

Subsequently, the ***mixed*** command is used for the first two visits as can be seen below:

```
mixed weight sport if visit < 3, || id:,  stddev
```

Output

```
Mixed-effects ML regression          Number of obs      =         40
Group variable: id                   Number of groups   =         20

                                     Obs per group:
                                                    min =          2
                                                    avg =        2.0
                                                    max =          2
                                     Wald chi2(1)       =      14.12
Log likelihood = -77.965175          Prob > chi2        =     0.0002
------------------------------------------------------------------------
```

```
  weight | Coef. Std. Err.      z  P>|z| [95% Conf. Interval]
---------+----------------------------------------------------------
   sport | -3.2  .8514694   -3.76 0.000 -4.868849  -1.531151
   _cons | 67.4  .6020798  111.95 0.000  66.21995   68.58005
---------+----------------------------------------------------------


----------------------------------------------------------------------
Random-effects Parameters|Estimate Std. Err. [95% Conf. Interval]
-------------------------+--------------------------------------------
id: Identity             |
            sd(_cons)    |1.746425 .3322952   1.202792   2.535768
-------------------------+--------------------------------------------
         sd(Residual)    | 1.07238 .1695582   .7866148    1.46196
----------------------------------------------------------------------
LR test vs. linear model: chibar2(01) = 14.99 Prob >= chibar2 = 0.0001
```

The results indicate that there is a significant change in the expected weight by sport (*P*-value <.001), even after controlling for the effect between subjects ($\hat{\beta}_1 = -3.2$ 95% CI: $-4.87, -1.53$). The intraclass correlation coefficient is determined with the following estimates:

$$\hat{\sigma}_{U_0} = 1.74$$

$$\hat{\sigma}_{\varepsilon} = 1.07$$

$$\hat{\rho} = \frac{1.74^2}{1.74^2 + 1.07^2} = .73$$

We can see that the average intercept is $\hat{\gamma}_{00} = 67.4$ and varies per visit ± 1.74.

Another option when running the mixed model with a random intercept is to use the ***gllamm*** command, which may be downloaded from www.gllamm.org. The result is the following, assuming that the data are in the long format:

```
gllamm weight sport if visit < 3, i(id) nip(20)
```

Output

```
gllamm model

log likelihood = -77.94849
```

```
weight |    Coef.   Std. Err.    z    P>|z|  [95% Conf.  Interval]
--------+-------------------------------------------------------
  sport |-3.194099 .8346379  -3.83 0.000   -4.829959  -1.558239
  _cons | 67.38501 .570114  118.20 0.000    66.26761   68.50241
--------------------------------------------------------------

Variance at level 1
--------------------------------------------------------------
 1.1368944 (.37024967)

Variances and covariances of random effects
--------------------------------------------------------------

***level 2 (id)

  var(1): 3.1128248 (1.2621798)
--------------------------------------------------------------
```

The results of both **mixed** and **gllamm** are similar, with a slight difference in the log-likelihood estimate and in the variance of random effects.

11.5 Using the *mixed* Command with Random Intercept and Slope

Another way to express a mixed model that explains the expected values of $Y(\mu_{ij})$ is to assume that the intercept and the slope are random variables, as follows:

$$\mu_{ij} = \beta_{0i} + \beta_{1i} * X_{ij}$$

where:
$\beta_{0i} = \gamma_{00} + U_{0i}$ (random coefficient)
β_{1i} indicates a random coefficient associated with the predictor X, which is defined as follows: $\gamma_{01} + U_{1i}$
$U_{0i} \sim N\left(0, \sigma_{U_0}^2\right)$
$U_{1i} \sim N\left(0, \sigma_{U_1}^2\right)$
γ_{00} indicates the average intercept in a design with two levels
γ_{01} indicates the average slope in a design with two levels
σ_{u0}^2 indicates the variance of the intercept between subjects
σ_{u1}^2 indicates the variance of the slope between subjects

In this mixed model, the variance of Y_{ij}, given X_{ij}, is enumerated by the following expression:

$$\text{var}\left(Y_{ij} \mid X_{ij}\right) = \sigma_{u0}^2 + 2\sigma_{01}X_{ij} + \sigma_{u1}^2 X_{ij}^2 + \sigma_\varepsilon^2,$$

where σ_{01} is the covariance between the intercept and the slope.

In addition, there is a possibility that there is a correlation between each of two different visits $(j \neq j')$ by the same subject, which is calculated from the covariance, as follows:

$$\text{Cov}\left(Y_{ij}, Y_{ij'} \mid X_{ij}, X_{ij'}\right) = \sigma_{u0}^2 + \sigma_{01}\left(X_{ij} + X_{ij'}\right) + \sigma_{u1}^2 * X_{ij} * X_{ij'}$$

As a consequence, the intraclass correlation coefficients with random intercept and random slope will be defined as follows:

$$\rho\left(Y_{ij} \mid X_{ij}\right) = \frac{\text{Cov}\left(Y_{ij}, Y_{ij'} \mid X_{ij}, X_{ij'}\right)}{\text{Var}\left(Y_{ij} \mid X_{ij}\right)} = \frac{\sigma_{u0}^2 + \sigma_{01}(X_{ij} + X_{ij'}) + \sigma_{u1}^2 X_{ij} * X_{ij'}}{\sigma_{u0}^2 + 2\sigma_{01}X_{ij} + \sigma_{u1}^2 X_{ij}^2 + \sigma_\varepsilon^2}$$

Therefore, this intraclass correlation coefficient will depend on the value of X.

When the intercept and slope are random in a mixed model, we can use the Stata command *mixed* with the previous database considering the three visits as follows:

```
mixed weight sport, || id: || sport:, stddev
```

Output

```
Mixed-effects ML regression              Number of obs    =      60
-------------------------------------------------------------
               | No. of    Observations per Group
Group Variable | Groups  Minimum  Average  Maximum
---------------+---------------------------------------------
           id  |   20        3       3.0       3
        sport  |   20        3       3.0       3
-------------------------------------------------------------

                                  Wald chi2(1)      =    5.16
Log likelihood = -140.95844       Prob > chi2       =  0.0231

-------------------------------------------------------------------
  weight |   Coef.   Std. Err.    z    P>|z|  [95% Conf. Interval]
---------+---------------------------------------------------------
   sport |-2.133333 .9387534  -2.27  0.023  -3.973256  -.2934105
   _cons | 66.43333 .6637989 100.08  0.000  65.13231   67.73436
-------------------------------------------------------------------
```

```
-----------------------------------------------------------------------
Random-effects Parameters |Estimate Std. Err. [95% Conf. Interval]
--------------------------+--------------------------------------------
id: Identity              |
             sd(_cons)    |1.206639 18.1424   1.92e-13   7.58e+12
--------------------------+--------------------------------------------
sport: Identity           |
             sd(_cons)    |1.206645 18.14232 1.92e-13   7.58e+12
--------------------------+--------------------------------------------
          sd(Residual)    |2.1173    .2367064 1.700675   2.635989
-----------------------------------------------------------------------
LR test vs. linear model: chi2(2) = 8.40 Prob > chi2 =  0.0150
```

The results indicate that there is a significant change in the average expected weight by sport (*P*-value = .023), even after controlling for the effect between subjects ($\hat{\gamma}_{01} = -2.13$, 95% CI: -3.97, -0.29). However, the average of the slopes associated with the sport predictor will vary ± 1.21, so the pattern of change in the average weight will depend on each visit.

11.6 Mixed Models in a Sampling Design

Let us assume that we have the following information from a random sample of 88 subjects, which will be used to assess the association between hepatitis C virus infection (hcv: 1 = present; 0 = absent) and cocaine metabolite assay result (co: 1 = positive; 0 = negative), controlling for the variables age (age2: 1 = <45 years; 2 = ≥45 years) and residential block (block), selected randomly:

```
     +-------------------------------+
     | block    co    hcv    age2    |
     |-------------------------------|
 1.  |   3      0      0      2      |
 2.  |   4      1      1      1      |
 3.  |   4      1      0      2      |
 4.  |   1      0      0      2      |
 5.  |   1      0      0      1      |
     |-------------------------------|
 6.  |   1      1      1      1      |
 7.  |   4      1      0      1      |
 8.  |   4      0      0      1      |
 9.  |   2      0      0      1      |
10.  |   2      0      0      1      |
     |-------------------------------|
11.  |   3      0      1      2      |
12.  |   2      0      0      1      |
13.  |   2      1      0      2      |
14.  |   4      0      0      1      |
15.  |   3      0      0      1      |
     |-------------------------------|
```

```
16. |    1    1    0    2 |
17. |    1    0    0    1 |
18. |    4    1    0    1 |
19. |    2    1    1    1 |
20. |    2    1    0    1 |
    |---------------------|
21. |    2    0    0    1 |
22. |    2    1    0    1 |
23. |    3    0    0    1 |
24. |    3    1    0    1 |
25. |    3    0    0    1 |
    |---------------------|
26. |    3    0    0    2 |
27. |    1    1    0    1 |
28. |    1    1    0    1 |
29. |    4    0    0    2 |
30. |    4    0    0    1 |
    |---------------------|
31. |    4    1    1    2 |
32. |    4    1    1    1 |
33. |    1    0    0    1 |
34. |    2    0    1    1 |
35. |    2    0    0    1 |
    |---------------------|
36. |    3    0    0    2 |
37. |    3    0    1    1 |
38. |    2    1    0    2 |
39. |    4    0    0    1 |
40. |    4    0    1    1 |
    |---------------------|
41. |    1    0    0    1 |
42. |    4    0    0    2 |
43. |    4    0    0    1 |
44. |    1    0    0    1 |
45. |    2    1    0    2 |
    |---------------------|
46. |    2    0    0    1 |
47. |    1    1    1    1 |
48. |    1    1    0    1 |
49. |    3    0    0    1 |
50. |    3    0    0    2 |
    |---------------------|
51. |    2    0    1    1 |
52. |    2    1    0    1 |
53. |    2    0    0    1 |
54. |    4    0    0    1 |
55. |    4    0    0    1 |
    |---------------------|
```

```
56. |     4      1      1      1 |
57. |     4      0      0      1 |
58. |     4      0      0      1 |
59. |     3      1      0      1 |
60. |     3      1      0      2 |
    |--------------------------|
61. |     3      1      0      1 |
62. |     4      1      1      2 |
63. |     2      0      0      1 |
64. |     2      0      0      1 |
65. |     2      0      0      2 |
    |--------------------------|
66. |     1      0      0      2 |
67. |     2      0      0      1 |
68. |     2      0      0      2 |
69. |     4      0      0      1 |
70. |     2      0      0      2 |
    |--------------------------|
71. |     2      1      0      1 |
72. |     2      1      0      2 |
73. |     2      0      0      2 |
74. |     2      0      0      1 |
75. |     2      0      0      1 |
    |--------------------------|
76. |     3      1      0      2 |
77. |     3      0      0      2 |
78. |     3      0      0      1 |
79. |     1      0      0      1 |
80. |     1      0      0      2 |
    |--------------------------|
81. |     1      0      0      2 |
82. |     3      1      0      2 |
83. |     1      1      0      2 |
84. |     1      0      0      2 |
85. |     2      1      0      1 |
    |--------------------------|
86. |     2      0      0      1 |
87. |     2      1      0      2 |
88. |     1      1      0      1 |
    +--------------------------+
```

If the data are analyzed under the assumption that there is a possible correlation between the subjects that reside in the same block (random intercept), the syntax of the *gllamm* command line to estimate the prevalence ratio using a logistic regression model with the option *link(log)*, which is called log-binomial regression model, is as follows:

```
xi:gllamm hcv i.co i.age2,fam(bin) i(block) eform link(log)
```

Output

```
gllamm model

log likelihood = -34.37179
```

```
--------------------------------------------------------------------------
      hcv | exp(b)    Std. Err.   z    P>|z|    [95% Conf. Interval]
----------+---------------------------------------------------------------
   _Ico_1 |2.834653 1.482238 1.99   0.046    1.017202    7.899373
 _Iage2_2 |.5385232 .3316394 -1.01  0.315     .1610675   1.800532
    _cons |.1036169 .0489457 -4.80  0.000     .0410533    .2615254
--------------------------------------------------------------------------
Variances and covariances of random effects
--------------------------------------------------------------------------

***level 2 (block)

   var(1): .0386266 (.20576199)
--------------------------------------------------------------------------
```

The results show that the prevalence of HCV infection among cocaine users is 2.83 (95% CI: 1.02, 7.90) times the prevalence of HCV infection among cocaine nonusers, adjusting for age and block of residence. This excess was statistically significant (*P*-value = .046).

There are other applications of multilevel modeling in health sciences that can be explored in Stata, including ordinal outcomes, count outcomes, and censored outcomes. These topics are beyond the scope of this book, but an extensive review of multilevel modeling can be found in Snijders and Bosker (2003), Leyland and Goldstein (2001), Twisk (2003), and Rabe-Hesketh and Skrondal (2005).

Chapter 12

Introduction to Advanced Programming in STATA

Aim: Upon completing the chapter, the learner should be able to develop short programs that will make the existing Stata commands run more efficiently.

12.1 Introduction

Stata provides an editor window to save Stata commands and user-defined commands. These files can be executed within this editor or they can be called for execution within another do-file. In this chapter, we will present an introduction about how to prepare do-files and the structure to define program commands (Juul, 2014).

12.2 do-files

The do-file editor tool can be used for data management and to create programs. There are four ways to open a new do-file: (1) the Windows menu (Window → do-file editor); (2) the keyboard (press Crtl+9); (3) the Windows icon (using the new do-file editor); and (4) using the command line *doedit*.

Example 1

Open a new do-file editor using the command window by typing "doedit." A do-file editor page will open. Create the following do-file:

```
noisily display "Introduction to STATA Programming"
noisily display "Example 1: New Do-file"
noisily display "END"
```

Then, save it under "\Users\Documents\students\example1.do."

To run the example1.do file, use the command window. To do this, you can type

```
cd "\Users\Documents\students"
do "example1.do",
```

and the following will appear:

```
. noisily display "Introduction to STATA Programming"
Introduction to STATA Programming
. noisily display "Example 1: New Do-file"
Example 1: New Do-file
. noisily display "END"
END
```

Or you can type

```
run example1,
```

and the following will appear:

```
Introduction to STATA Programming
Example 1: New Do-file
END
```

The commands ***noisily*** and ***quietly*** are special commands that turn the output on and off. The first, ***noisily***, performs the command subsequently written and ensures terminal output. The second, ***quietly***, performs the command subsequently written but suppresses terminal output. As you can see in the example above, if you type "do" before typing "example1," all the information in the do-file will be displayed in the Stata results window. If you type "run," only the information after the ***noisily display*** commands will be shown in the output window.

12.3 *program* Command

The *program* command is used to do data management and to run analyses. The following is the basic structure to use the program command:

```
program program name
{a series of STATA commands}
end
```

When you are writing a program, the program name has to be unique and cannot be the same as any other command name. For example, you cannot use the name "ttest" because it is a built-in command in Stata. To be able to find out whether a name is already in use by Stata, you can use the *which* command. In the command window type *which program name*. Doing so will result in the following:

```
. which ttest
C:\Program Files (x86)\Stata\ado\base\t\ttest.ado
*! version 4.1.1  30dec2004
. which example
command example not found as either built-in or ado-file
r(111);
```

As you can see in the previous example, a program named "ttest" is being used by Stata, and the program name "example" is not being used. *Example2.do* illustrates the use of the *program* command using the command window. Type the following lines in the command field:

```
program example2
display "Example 2: How to use the command program"
display "STATA commands"
display "End of the Example"
end
```

To execute the program, type "example2" in the command line; the output after having done so will be:

```
Example 2: How to use the command program
STATA commands
End of the Example
```

If you want to change or edit a program, you will need to first delete that program from the memory. If you try to use the name "example2" again, you will get the following error:

```
program example2
example3 already defined
r(110);
```

To delete this error or cause it to be ignored, you can use the commands *drop* and *capture*. The *drop* command deletes the program from the memory, and the *capture* command causes the errors associated with the command that follows the *capture* command to be ignored. Type the following example in the command line, or create a do-file with these commands:

```
capture program drop example3
program example3
display "Example 3: How to use the commands drop and capture"
display "STATA commands"
display "End of the Example"
end
```

Then, type "example3" in the command window.

```
Example 3: How to use the commands drop and capture
STATA commands
End of the Example
```

12.4 Log Files

It is important to keep track of your work while you are programming. If you keep a log of your work, you will find it easier to go back and check what you have already done. To create a log, use the following steps:

1. To start:
   Menu toolbar → File – Log – Begin → Save as *filename*
2. To finish:
   Menu toolbar → File – Log – Close

Or, write the following in the command window:

```
log using "C:\MyPrograms\mylog", replace
{a series of STATA commands and their outputs}
log close
```

For example, prepare a do-file, named "example4," as follows:

```
log using "example4", replace text
use "/Users/Documents/bmi.dta"
tab bmig
```

bmig	Freq.	Percent	Cum.
Normal	4	40.00	40.00
Overweight	3	30.00	70.00
Obese	3	30.00	100.00
Total	10	100.00	

```
log close
```

After *log using* command, all the commands and their outputs will be saved in example4.txt until *log close* command.

12.5 *trace* Command

While you are programming, sometimes you will get errors after executing a given program. The *trace* command is a useful tool for finding these errors. You can turn this command on or off at any time while you are programming. The following do-file, named "example5," illustrates how to use the *trace* command:

```
capture log close

log using "example5.log", replace
```

```
capture program drop _all
 program example5
      display "Example #5"
      display "Runs the error when you run the program"
      display "Stops and displays the error when executing the
      program"
      display "End of the Example"
      ERRORRRRRR
 end
log close
set trace on
set more off
example5
```

If you run the do-file named "example5," you will get the following error:

```
. example5
---------------------------------------- begin example5 ---
- display "Example #5"
Example #5
- display "Runs the error when you run the program"
Runs the error when you run the program
- display "Stops and displays the error when executing the
program"
Stops and displays the error when executing the program
- display "End of the Example"
End of the Example
- ERRORRRRRR
unrecognized command:  ERRORRRRRR
---------------------------------------- end example5 ---
r(199);
end of do-file
```

12.6 Delimiters

Stata reads each line as a complete command line, but sometimes the commands are long. To be able to use more than one line as your command line you can use delimiters. There are two types of delimiters, one you can use in each line (*///*), and one you set up before running your Stata commands (*#d ;*). The following examples show how each of the two delimiters is used to create a two-way graph:

```
twoway (scatter bmi age if sex==0, sort mcolor(navy)              ///
        msymbol(circle_hollow))                                  ///
      (scatter bmi age if sex==1, sort mcolor(maroon)   msymbol(circle)) ///
      (line    bmi age if sex==0, sort lcolor(navy)    lwidth(thick)) ///
```

```
(line     bmi age if sex==1, sort lcolor(maroon) lwidth(thick)),///
legend(position(10) ring(0) col(1) order(1 "Males" 2 "Females")///
region(fcolor(none) lcolor(none)))                              ///
ylab(, angle(horizontal)) ytitle("BMI") xtitle("Age") graphregion(fcolor
(white))
```

And

```
#d ;
twoway (scatter bmi age if sex==0, sort mcolor(navy)  msymbol(circle_hollow))
(scatter bmi age if sex==1,    sort mcolor(maroon) msymbol(circle))
(line      bmi age if sex==0,    sort lcolor(navy)    lwidth(thick))
(line      bmi age if sex==1,    sort lcolor(maroon) lwidth(thick)),
legend(position(10) ring(0) col(1) order(1 "Males" 2 "Females")
region(fcolor(none) lcolor(none))) ylab( , angle(horizontal))
ytitle("BMI") xtitle("Age") graphregion(fcolor(white));
#d cr
```

As you can see above, you need to open with **#d ;** and then close with **#d cr** for the next command lines. If you do not close the delimiter, Stata will continue to read all the lines continuously.

12.7 Indexing

When you execute a Stata command, the command will loop across each line of the dataset. For example, if you generate a new variable, Stata will work in line 1, then line 2, and so on. The use of indexing will help the user to run only Stata commands in certain observations. The following are examples of indexing:

1. Generate a new variable, *x*, that contains the number of the current observation:

   ```
   gen x=_n
   ```

   Output

   ```
   . list x

        +---+
        | x |
        |---|
     1. | 1 |
     2. | 2 |
     3. | 3 |
     4. | 4 |
     5. | 5 |
        |---|
     6. | 6 |
     7. | 7 |
        +---+
   ```

2. Generate a new variable, *y*, which contains the total number of observations in the dataset, assuming the last dataset:

```
gen y=_N
```

. list x y

```
     +-------+
     | x   y |
     |-------|
1.   | 1   7 |
2.   | 2   7 |
3.   | 3   7 |
4.   | 4   7 |
5.   | 5   7 |
     |-------|
6.   | 6   7 |
7.   | 7   7 |
     +-------+
```

3. To check for duplicates in your dataset, assuming every subject has an id, which is identified in this dataset by ID and it is a sequential set of numbers starting with 1, use the following command line:

```
bysort ID: gen duplicates = _n
```

4. To create a variable with the total number of subjects in a group, where these groups are identified by *groupid*, use the following command line:

```
bysort groupid: gen subjects = _N
```

5. Generate two new variables, *z* and *w*. Variable *z* contains the current observation minus 1. The first observation will be missing. Variable *w* contains the current observation plus 1. The last observation will be missing. Observe:

```
gen z=x[_n-1]
gen w=x[_n+1]
```

list x y z w

```
     +-----------------+
     | x   y   z   w |
     |-----------------|
1.   | 1   7   .   2 |
2.   | 2   7   1   3 |
3.   | 3   7   2   4 |
4.   | 4   7   3   5 |
5.   | 5   7   4   6 |
6.   | 6   7   5   7 |
7.   | 7   7   6   . |
     +-----------------+
```

12.8 Local Macros

Local macros are temporary variables in the memory for loops and programs. A local macro can be a number or a string of characters (in either case, up to 31 characters can be used). To exemplify these macros, let's assume the following database:

```
. list
```

```
     +-------------------------------+
     |  age   bmi    hgb   smoke |
     |-------------------------------|
 1.  |   18    18   11.3       1 |
 2.  |   19    24     14       1 |
 3.  |   23    27   14.5       1 |
 4.  |   25    24   14.7       0 |
 5.  |   37    28     15       0 |
     |-------------------------------|
 6.  |   56    29     13       0 |
 7.  |   78    32     12       0 |
 8.  |   52    23     11       1 |
 9.  |   21    24     14       1 |
10.  |   45    20   11.5       1 |
     |-------------------------------|
11.  |   25    24   14.7       0 |
12.  |   34    20     12       0 |
13.  |   59    29     13       0 |
14.  |   78    32     12       0 |
     +-------------------------------+
```

If we are interested in using age and hemoglobin (hgb) levels as predictors of bmi, we could define the list of predictors and then run a multivariate linear regression model, as follows:

```
local list = "age hgb"
reg bmi 'list'
```

Output

```
  Source |       SS          df       MS          Number of obs  =      14
---------+----------------------------------      F(2, 11)       =   43.77
   Model | 221.078339        2   110.539169       Prob > F       =  0.0000
Residual |  27.7788042       11  2.52534584       R-squared      =  0.8884
---------+----------------------------------      Adj R-squared  =  0.8681
   Total | 248.857143        13  19.1428571       Root MSE       =  1.5891

-----------------------------------------------------------------------------
     bmi |    Coef.    Std. Err.      t     P>|t|     [95% Conf. Interval]
---------+-------------------------------------------------------------------
     age |  .2179857   .0239641     9.10    0.000     .165241     .2707304
     hgb |  2.241635   .3550485     6.31    0.000    1.460178    3.023091
   _cons | -12.84275   5.193205    -2.47    0.031   -24.27292   -1.412584
-----------------------------------------------------------------------------
```

12.9 Scalars

Scalars are temporary results that are saved in the memory after a command is run. After you run a command, you can review which scalars were saved using the *return list* command. For example, let's assume that we have the variable *smoke* from the previous database, and we want to run a Student's *t*-test to compare the expected bmi by smoke. The following is what that would look like:

```
ttest bmi, by(smoke)
```

Output

```
Two-sample t test with equal variances
-----------------------------------------------------------------------------
  Group |    Obs       Mean    Std. Err.   Std. Dev.   [95% Conf.   Interval]
--------+--------------------------------------------------------------------
      0 |      8      27.25    1.497021    4.234214    23.71011    30.78989
      1 |      6   22.66667    1.308094    3.204164    19.3041     26.02923
--------+--------------------------------------------------------------------
combined |     14   25.28571    1.169336    4.375255    22.75952    27.81191
--------+--------------------------------------------------------------------
   diff |           4.583333    2.07317                .0662847    9.100382
-----------------------------------------------------------------------------
    diff = mean(0) - mean(1)                                 t =    2.2108
Ho: diff = 0                                  degrees of freedom =       12

    Ha: diff < 0              Ha: diff != 0              Ha: diff > 0
 Pr(T < t) = 0.9764     Pr(|T| > |t|) = 0.0472      Pr(T > t) = 0.0236
```

After Student's *t*-test, we use the *return* command, as follows:

```
return list
```

After doing so, the following results should appear:

```
scalars:
              r(level) =   95
                 r(sd) =   4.375255094603872
               r(sd_2) =   3.204163957519444
               r(sd_1) =   4.234214381508266
                 r(se) =   2.073169652345752
                r(p_u) =   .0236068853559555
                r(p_l) =   .9763931146440445
                  r(p) =   .047213770711911
                  r(t) =   2.210785464733855
               r(df_t) =   12
               r(mu_2) =   22.6666666666667
                r(N_2) =   6
               r(mu_1) =   27.25
                r(N_1) =   8
```

Scalars are useful for displaying only the results you want, instead of displaying all the results. Here is an example:

```
. noisily display "Pr(|T| > |t|) =" %9.3f `r(p)'
Pr(|T| > |t|) =      0.047
```

In addition, you can create new scalars to calculate results not included in the saved results. In the following example, using the previous database, the mean difference between two groups is calculated:

```
capture program drop example6
program example6, rclass
  summarize `1' if `2'==0, meanonly
  scalar mean1 = r(mean)
  summarize `1' if `2'==1, meanonly
  scalar mean2 = r(mean)
  return scalar diff = mean1 - mean2
end
```

After running the program named "example6," the following is returned:

```
. example6 bmi smoke

. return list

scalars:

r(diff) =   4.583333333333332
```

12.10 Loops (*foreach* and *forvalues*)

The command *foreach* repeatedly executes the commands enclosed inside the braces, as can be seen in the following:

```
foreach lname {in|of listtype} list {
commands referring to `lname'
}
```

Here is an example that uses the previous database with the following do-file:

```
foreach var of var bmi age hgb {
mean `var'
}
```

Output

```
Mean estimation                    Number of obs    =         14
--------------------------------------------------------------------
             |        Mean    Std. Err.      [95% Conf. Interval]
-------------+------------------------------------------------------
         bmi |    25.28571    1.169336       22.75952    27.81191
--------------------------------------------------------------------


Mean estimation                    Number of obs    =         14

--------------------------------------------------------------------
             |        Mean    Std. Err.      [95% Conf. Interval]
-------------+------------------------------------------------------
         age |    40.71429    5.614374       28.58517     52.8434
--------------------------------------------------------------------


Mean estimation                    Number of obs    =         14

--------------------------------------------------------------------
             |        Mean    Std. Err.      [95% Conf. Interval]
-------------+------------------------------------------------------
         hgb |       13.05    .3789444       12.23134    13.86866
--------------------------------------------------------------------
```

In addition, you can use the *local* command in the do-file, as can be seen in the following:

```
local variables = "bmi age hgb"
foreach var of local variables {
sum `var'
}
```

After doing so, the following results will appear:

```
    Variable |        Obs        Mean    Std. Dev.       Min        Max
-------------+--------------------------------------------------------
         bmi |         14    25.28571    4.375255        18         32

    Variable |        Obs        Mean    Std. Dev.       Min        Max
-------------+--------------------------------------------------------
         age |         14    40.71429    21.00706        18         78

    Variable |        Obs        Mean    Std. Dev.       Min        Max
-------------+--------------------------------------------------------
         hgb |         14       13.05     1.41788        11         15
```

The command *forvalues* loops over consecutive values, using the following structure:

```
forvalues lname = range {
commands referring to `lname'
}
```

For example, assuming we want to generate two random variables with uniform distribution between the numbers 1 and 14, and assuming we are using the previous bmi database, the do-file will be composed of the following commands:

```
forvalues i = 1(1)2  {
generate x`i' = 1+ int(runiform()*14)
}
```

Once the above *forvalues* command is run, the variables *x*1 and *x*2 are generated. To explore the values of these variables, we use *list*, as is demonstrated in the following:

```
. list x1 x2

     +-----------+
     |  x1    x2 |
     |-----------|
  1. |   7    13 |
  2. |  11    13 |
  3. |  13    11 |
  4. |   2    13 |
  5. |   7    10 |
     |-----------|
  6. |  13     4 |
  7. |  11    12 |
  8. |   4     1 |
  9. |   3    13 |
 10. |  11     5 |
     |-----------|
 11. |  14    11 |
 12. |  11     9 |
 13. |  13     5 |
 14. |   4     3 |
     +-----------+
```

Assuming we would like to select those persons for whom *x*1 is greater than *x*2 for further assessment, we would use the following commands:

```
gen id=_n
gen selec=(x1 > x2)
list id age bmi hgb smoke if selec==1
```

Output

```
+------------------------------------+
|  id   age   bmi    hgb   smoke |
|------------------------------------|
 3. |   3    23    27   14.5       1 |
 6. |   6    56    29     13       0 |
 8. |   8    52    23     11       1 |
10. |  10    45    20   11.5       1 |
11. |  11    25    24   14.7       0 |
|------------------------------------|
12. |  12    34    20     12       0 |
13. |  13    59    29     13       0 |
14. |  14    78    32     12       0 |
+------------------------------------+
```

Therefore, the individuals to be selected will be those with id*s* 3,6,8,10,11,12,13, and 14.

12.11 Application of *matrix* and *local* Commands for Prevalence Estimation

If we want to estimate the prevalence of one particular event, there are different Stata commands for performing this process, which include *proportion* and *glm*. The *proportion* command uses a normal approach (Rosner, 2010), and the *glm* command uses a logistic regression model (Hosmer and Lemeshow, 2000). For example, assuming we are interested in estimating the prevalence of women from the previous database who have a hemoglobin level below 12, the syntaxes with the *proportion* command will be as follows:

```
gen nhgb=hgb < 12
proportion nhgb
```

Output

```
Proportion estimation          Number of obs    =        14
----------------------------------------------------------------
            |  Proportion    Std. Err.      [95% Conf. Interval]
------------+---------------------------------------------------
nhgb        |
         0  |   .7857143     .1138039       .4598449    .9404495
         1  |   .2142857     .1138039       .0595505    .5401551
----------------------------------------------------------------
```

The prevalence estimate of a hemoglobin level below 12 is 21.4% (95% CI: 5.9, 54.0%).

If we want to use the *glm* command for this estimation, we will use the logistic regression model with no predictor variables, as follows:

$$\text{Prevalence} = \frac{1}{1+e^{-\beta_0}}$$

where β_0 is the intercept. The syntaxes for a prevalence estimate of hemoglobin levels below 12, after running the *glm* command, will be based on the *matrix* and *local* commands and are seen in the following:

```
quietly: glm nhgb , fam(bin)
matrix def b=e(b)
matrix def v=e(V)
local c=b[1,1]
local es=sqrt(v[1,1])
gen prev=100/(1+exp(-'c'))
gen previnf=100/(1+exp(-('c'-1.96*'es')))
gen prevsup=100/(1+exp(-('c'+1.96*'es')))
collapse (mean) prev previnf prevsup
list
```

The output of the above will be:

```
     +------------------------------------+
     |     prev     previnf     prevsup   |
     |------------------------------------|
  1. | 21.42857    7.070517    49.43356   |
     +------------------------------------
```

The point estimates of this prevalence are the same, but the confidence limits are different, probably because of the small sample size for the normal approach used in the *proportion* command.

The other option for prevalence estimation is to use the *adjust* command after the *logit* command, as is demonstrated in the following:

```
logit nhgb
adjust ,pr ci
```

Output

```
Logistic regression                 Number of obs   =          14
                                     LR chi2(0)      =        0.00
                                     Prob > chi2     =           .
Log likelihood = -7.2741177          Pseudo R2       =      0.0000
```

```
----------------------------------------------------------------------
nhgb |   Coef.    Std. Err.   z    P>|z|   [95% Conf. Interval]
---------+------------------------------------------------------------
_cons |  -1.299283 .6513389  -1.99 0.046   -2.575884   -.0226821
----------------------------------------------------------------------

. adjust ,pr ci

----------------------------------------------------------------------
Dependent variable: nhgb   Equation: nhgb      Command: logit
----------------------------------------------------------------------


---------------------------------------------------
All |            pr          lb          ub
-------+-------------------------------------------
    |        .214286    [.070707    .49433]
---------------------------------------------------

Key:  pr         =   Probability
     [lb , ub]   =   [95% Confidence Interval]
```

The results are the same as those obtained with the *glm* command. That is, the prevalence estimate of hemoglobin levels below 12 is 21.4% (95% CI: 7.07%, 49.43%).

When the logistic regression model includes predictors, prevalence estimation can be performed setting the value of only one of the predictors. For example, if we run the previous logistic model with *age* as the predictor, the prevalence can be estimated at *mean bmi* and at *bmi equal to 20,* as follows:

```
logit nhgb bmi
adjust , pr ci
adjust bmi=20, pr ci
```

Output

```
Logistic regression                     Number of obs   =         14
                                         LR chi2(1)      =       7.09
                                         Prob > chi2     =     0.0078
Log likelihood = -3.729784               Pseudo R2       =     0.4873


----------------------------------------------------------------------
nhgb |   Coef.    Std. Err.   z    P>|z|   [95% Conf. Interval]
---------+------------------------------------------------------------
 bmi |  -.7007166  .4025497  -1.74 0.082   -1.489699   .0882662
_cons |  14.81156   8.899236  1.66 0.096   -2.630626   32.25374
----------------------------------------------------------------------

. adjust , pr ci
```

```
------------------------------------------------------------------------------
      Dependent variable: nhgb      Equation: nhgb      Command: logit
      Variable left as is: bmi
------------------------------------------------------------------------------


     ---------------------------------------------------
        All |          pr           lb           ub
     -----------+---------------------------------------
            |      .05183      [.00225      .569917]
     ---------------------------------------------------

      Key:  pr          =  Probability
            [lb , ub]   =  [95% Confidence Interval]

.  adjust bmi=20, pr ci


------------------------------------------------------------------------------
      Dependent variable: nhgb      Equation: nhgb      Command: logit
 Covariate set to value: bmi = 20
------------------------------------------------------------------------------


     ---------------------------------------------------
        All |          pr           lb           ub
     -----------+---------------------------------------
            |      .68938      [.165612      .961265]
     ---------------------------------------------------

      Key:  pr          =  Probability
            [lb , ub]   =  [95% Confidence Interval]
```

The prevalence estimate of hemoglobin levels below 12 set at mean bmi is 5.2% (95% CI: 0.22%, 57.0%). The prevalence estimate of hemoglobin levels below 12 for those subjects with bmi equal to 20 is 68.9% (95% CI: 16.56%, 96.13%). Although the bmi predictor in the model is marginally significant (*P*-value = .082), the prevalence estimates at different bmi values are quite different.

There are other options of programming that can be explored in Stata, including different procedures for matrix operations using *Mata* functions. These topics are beyond the scope of this book, so we recommend checking out the books by Acock (*A Gentle Introduction to Stata,* 4th edition, 2014) and by Baum (*An Introduction to Stata Programming,* 2009).

References

Acock A. *A Gentle Introduction to Stata*. 4th ed. College Station, TX: Stata Press, 2014.

Baum C. *An Introduction to Stata Programming*. College Station, TX: Stata Press, 2009.

Bingham N, Fry J. *Regression Linear Models in Statistics*. London, UK: Springer-Verlag, 2010.

Cameron A, Trivedi P. *Regression Analysis of Count Data*. London, UK: Cambridge University Press, 1998.

Collett D. *Modelling Binary Data*. 2nd ed. London: Chapman & Hall, 2002.

Collett D. *Modelling Survival Data in Medical Research*. 2nd ed. London, UK: Chapman & Hall, 2003.

Draper NR, Smith H. *Applied Regression Analysis*. 3rd ed. Hoboken, NJ: John Wiley & Sons, 1998.

Fox J. *Applied Regression Analysis and Generalized Linear Models*. 2nd ed. Thousand Oaks, CA: Sage Publications, 2008.

Fu J, Gao J, Zhang Z, Zheng J, Luo JF, Zhong LP, Xiang YB. Tea consumption and the risk of oral cancer incidence: A case-control study from China. *Oral Oncol*. 2013; 49:918–922.

Good PI. *Resampling Methods: A Practical Guide to Data Analysis*. 3rd ed. Boston, MA: Birkhäuser Basel, 2006.

Hardin J, Hilbe J. *Generalized Linear Models and Extensions*. 1st ed. College Station, TX: Stata Press, 2001.

Hilbe J. *Negative Binomial Regression*. New York: Cambridge University Press, 2007.

Hoffmann J. *Generalized Linear Models: An Applied Approach*. Boston, MA: Pearson/Allyn & Bacon, 2004.

Hosmer D, Lemeshow S. *Applied Logistic Regression*. 2nd ed. Hoboken, NJ: John Wiley & Sons, 2000.

Jewell N. *Statistics for Epidemiology*. Boca Raton, FL: Chapman & Hall, 2004.

Juul S, Frydenberg M. *An Introduction to STATA for Health Researchers*. 4th ed. College Station, TX: Stata Press, 2014.

Kleinbaum D, Klein M. *Logistic Regression: A Self-Learning Text*. 2nd ed. New York: Springer-Verlag, 2002.

Kleinbaum D, Klein M. *Survival Analysis: A Self-Learning Text*. 2nd ed. New York: Springer-Verlag, 2005.

Kleinbaum D, Kupper L, Nizam A, Muller K. *Applied Regression Analysis and Other Multivariable Methods*. 4th ed. Belmont, CA: Thomson Brooks, 2008.

Leyland A, Goldstein H. *Multilevel Modelling of Health Statistics*. Chichester: John Wiley & Sons, 2001.

Marschener I. *Inference Principles for Biostatisticians*. Boca Raton, FL: CRC Press, 2015.

McCullagh P, Nelder J. *Generalized Linear Models.* 2nd ed. Boca Raton, FL: Chapman & Hall, 1999.

Peace K (ed). *Design and Analysis of Clinical Trials with Time-to-Event Endpoints.* Boca Raton, FL: CRC Press, 2009.

Porta M (ed). *A Dictionary of Epidemiology.* 5th ed. New York: Oxford University Press, 2008.

Rabe-Hesketh S, Everitt B. *A Handbook of Statistical Analyses Using STATA.* Boca Raton, FL: Chapman & Hall, 1999.

Rabe-Hesketh S, Skrondal A. *Multilevel and Longitudinal Modeling Using STATA.* College Station, TX: Stata Press, 2005.

Rosner B. *Fundamentals of Biostatistics.* 7th ed. Boston, MA: Cengage Learning, 2010.

Rothman K. *Epidemiology: An Introduction.* New York: Oxford University Press, 2002.

Royston P, Lambert P. *Flexible Parametric Survival Analysis Using STATA: Beyond the Cox Model.* College Station, TX: Stata Press, 2011.

Sheskin D. *Handbook of Parametric and Nonparametric Statistical Procedures.* 4th ed. Boca Raton, FL: Chapman & Hall, 2007.

Snijder T, Bosker R. *Multilevel Analysis: An Introduction to Basic and Advanced Multilevel Modeling.* Thousand Oaks, CA: Sage Publications, 1999, reprinted 2003.

Szklo M, Nieto J. *Epidemiology: Beyond the Basics.* Sudbury, MA: Jones and Bartlett, 2004.

Twisk J. *Applied Longitudinal Data Analysis for Epidemiology: A Practical Guide.* London, UK: Cambridge University Press, 2003.

Wienke A. *Frailty Models in Survival Analysis.* Boca Raton, FL: CRC Press, 2011.

Woodward M. *Epidemiology: Study Design and Data Analysis.* 2nd ed. Boca Raton, FL: Chapman & Hall, 2004.

Index